# Breaking Free

## Coloring Book Therapy for Addiction & Recovery

### by April McCallum

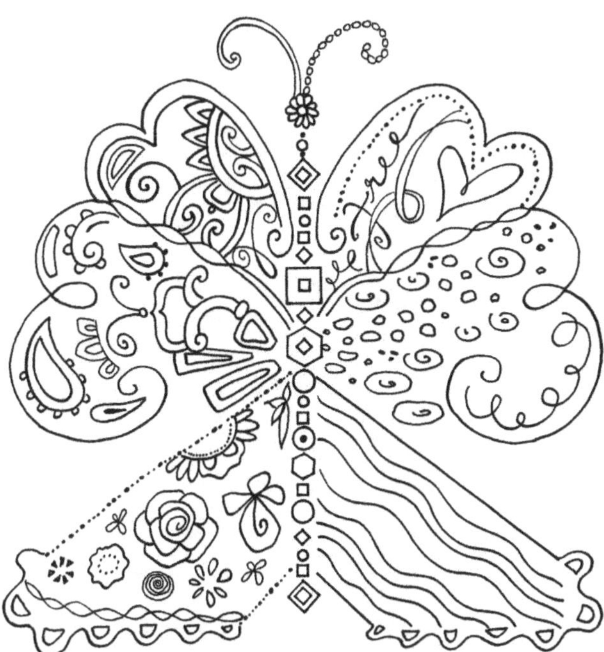

ISBN: 978-1-7325752-1-9

**Breaking Free:** Coloring Book Therapy for Addiction & Recovery
(c) 2019 by April McCallum
Published in the United States by Heart & Key Publishing

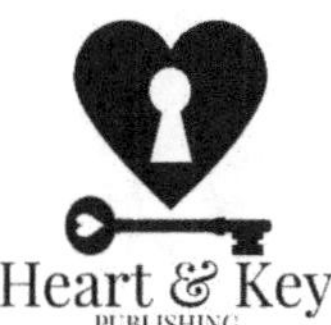


Cover Design Collaboration and Colorization by Pete Berg
www.aprilmccallumdesigns.com

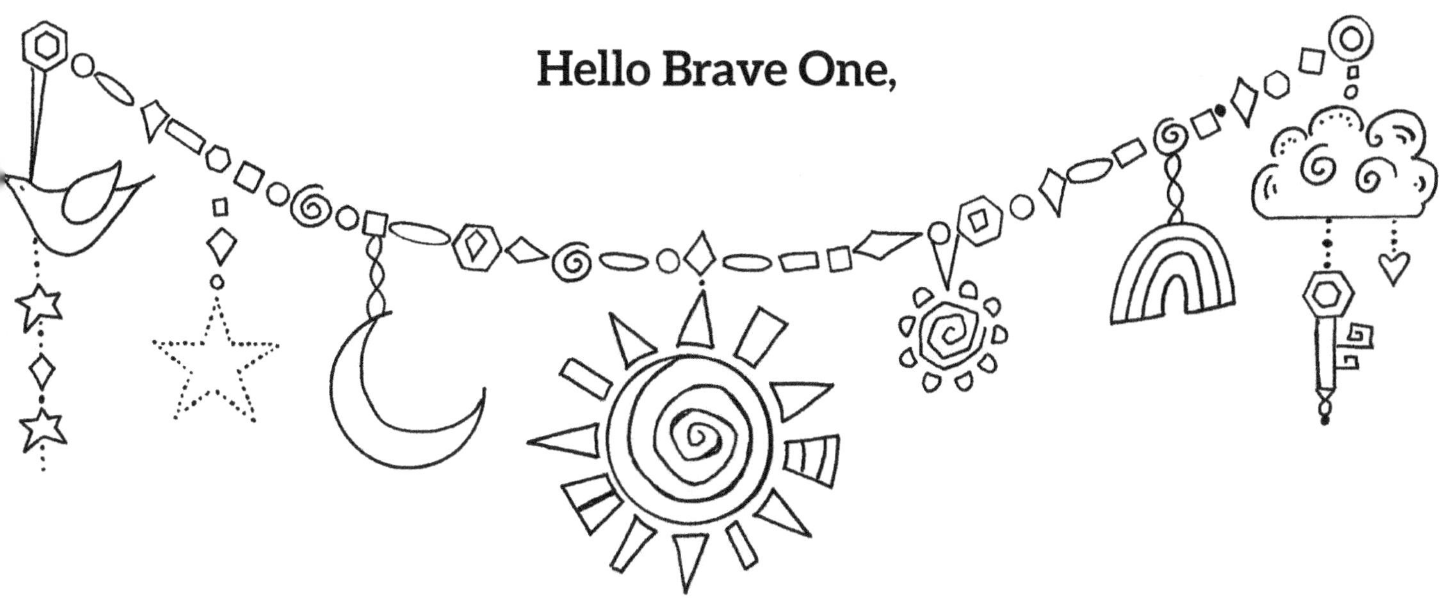

# Hello Brave One,

**Art and Heart...** I'm so happy you are here! Breaking Free is a collection of coloring pages that was created with love, just for you. This coloring book was designed to be a positive, truth-charged, hope-filled and empowering companion for those connected with the ever-challenging struggle and complexity of addiction.

*Breaking Free* is a powerful combination of beautiful hand (and heart) drawn illustrations, thoughts and quotes to encourage you on your journey to recovery. May it inspire you to break free and live your best life now. Art Buchwald said, "Whether it's the best of times or the worst of times, it's the only time we've got." Life. No one said it would be easy, but when we're free — *really free* — we find the process of sprouting wings was so worth it! Be kind to yourself. Keep looking up. Keep moving forward. One step in front of the next. And when you can finally breathe free, lift someone else and encourage them to do the same. Nothing feels as beautiful as freedom. Nothing is as intoxicating as living the life that we were made for.

> *"Even in the midst of devastation, something within us*
> *always points the way to freedom." — Sharon Salzberg*

Tips: If you would like to practice your lines and coloring tools, you will find a blank page in the back of the book to do just that. If you plan to use non-dry coloring materials, please place a blank sheet or two under the page you're coloring so it doesn't bleed through.

Consider this book a place for you to rest, meditate and recharge as you color.

Here's to breaking free and living free!

XO
*April*

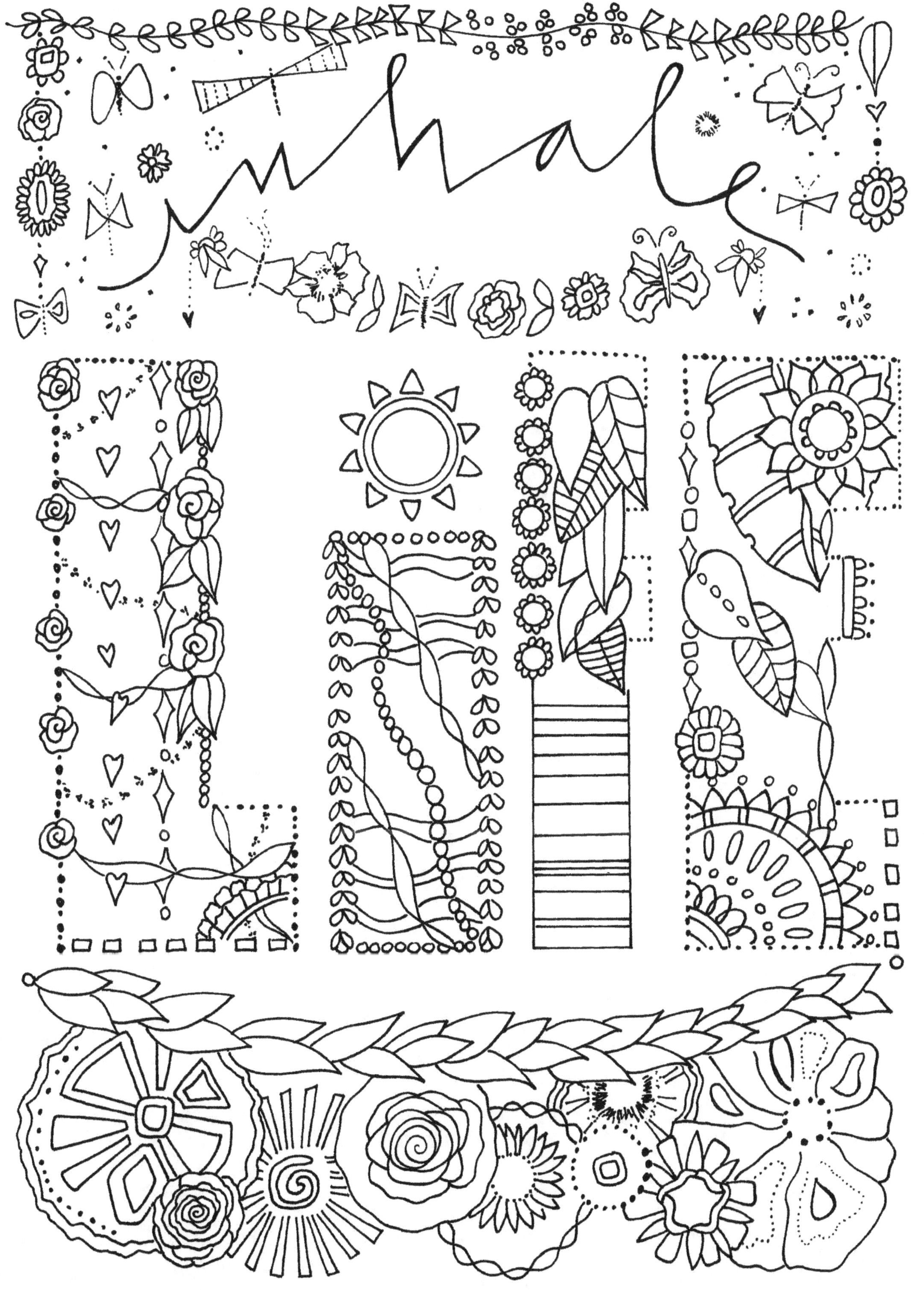

Inhale

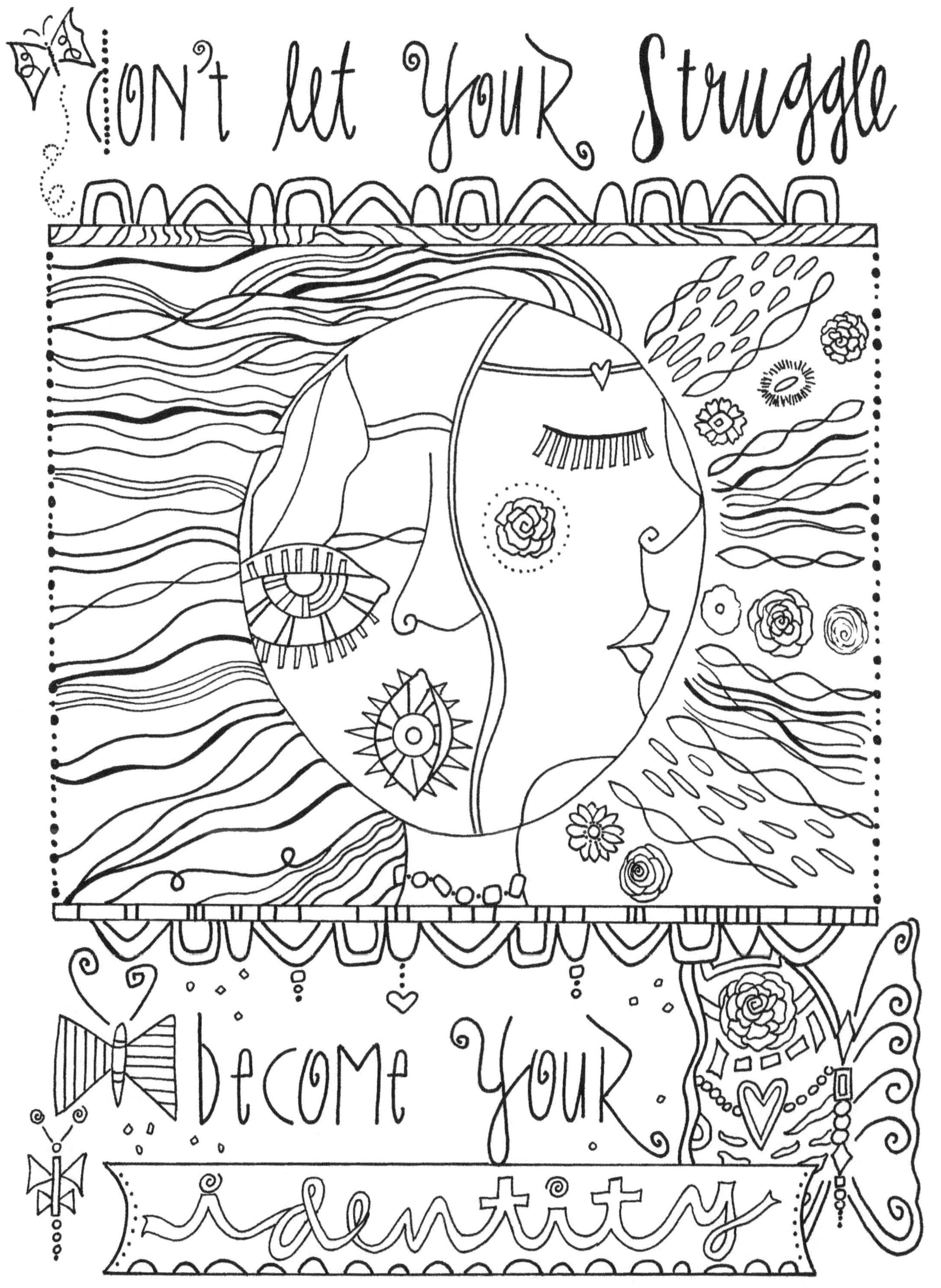
Don't let your Struggle
become Your
identity

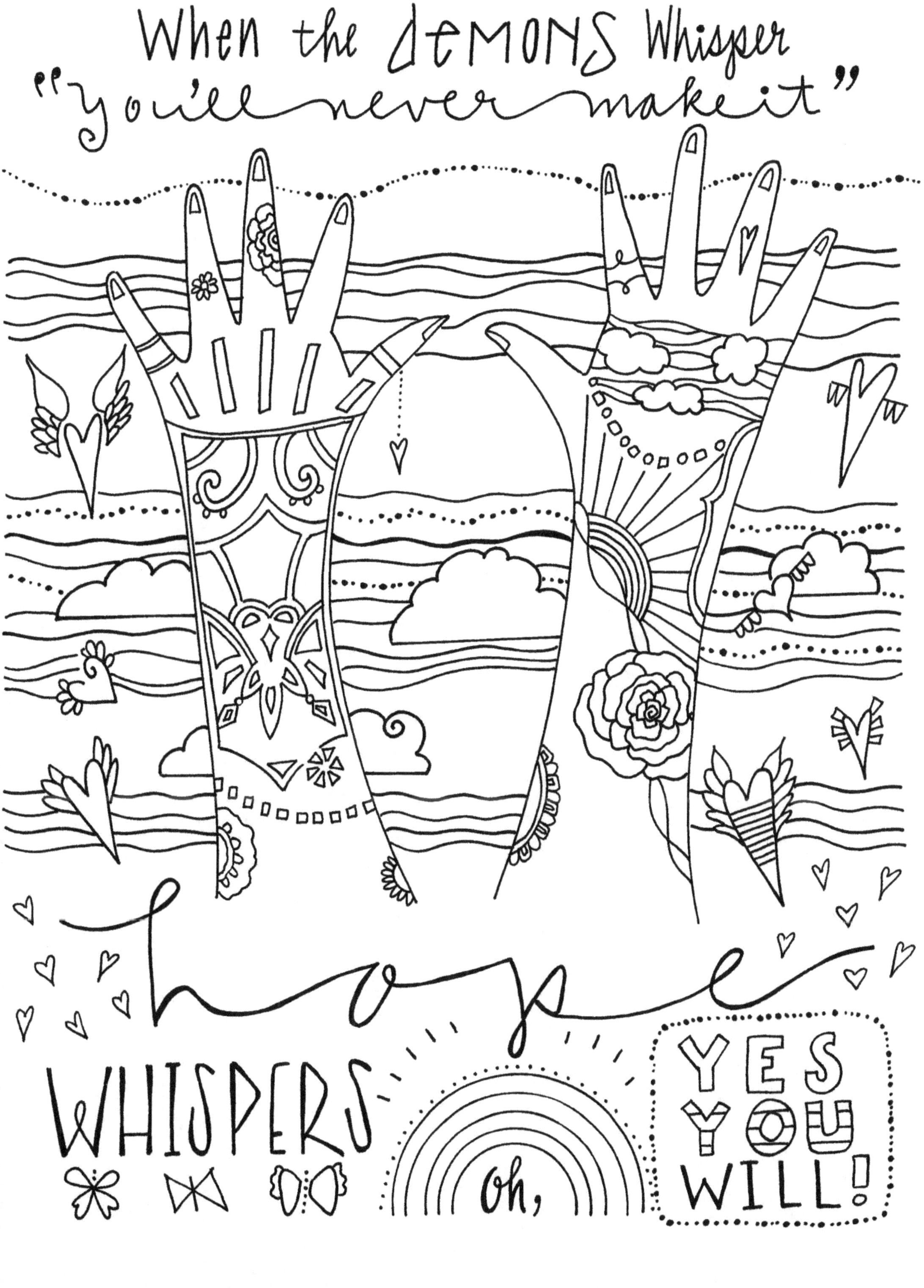

When the DEMONS Whisper
"You'll never make it"

hope

WHISPERS

Oh,

YES YOU WILL!

Happiness

when you can have the Real thing.

Never settle for the illusion of

Fantasies don't LOVE you back.

You are not the victim of the world, but rather the master of your own destiny. It is your choices & decisions that determine your destiny. Roy bennett

PEOPLE are NOT addicted to alcohol or DRUGS

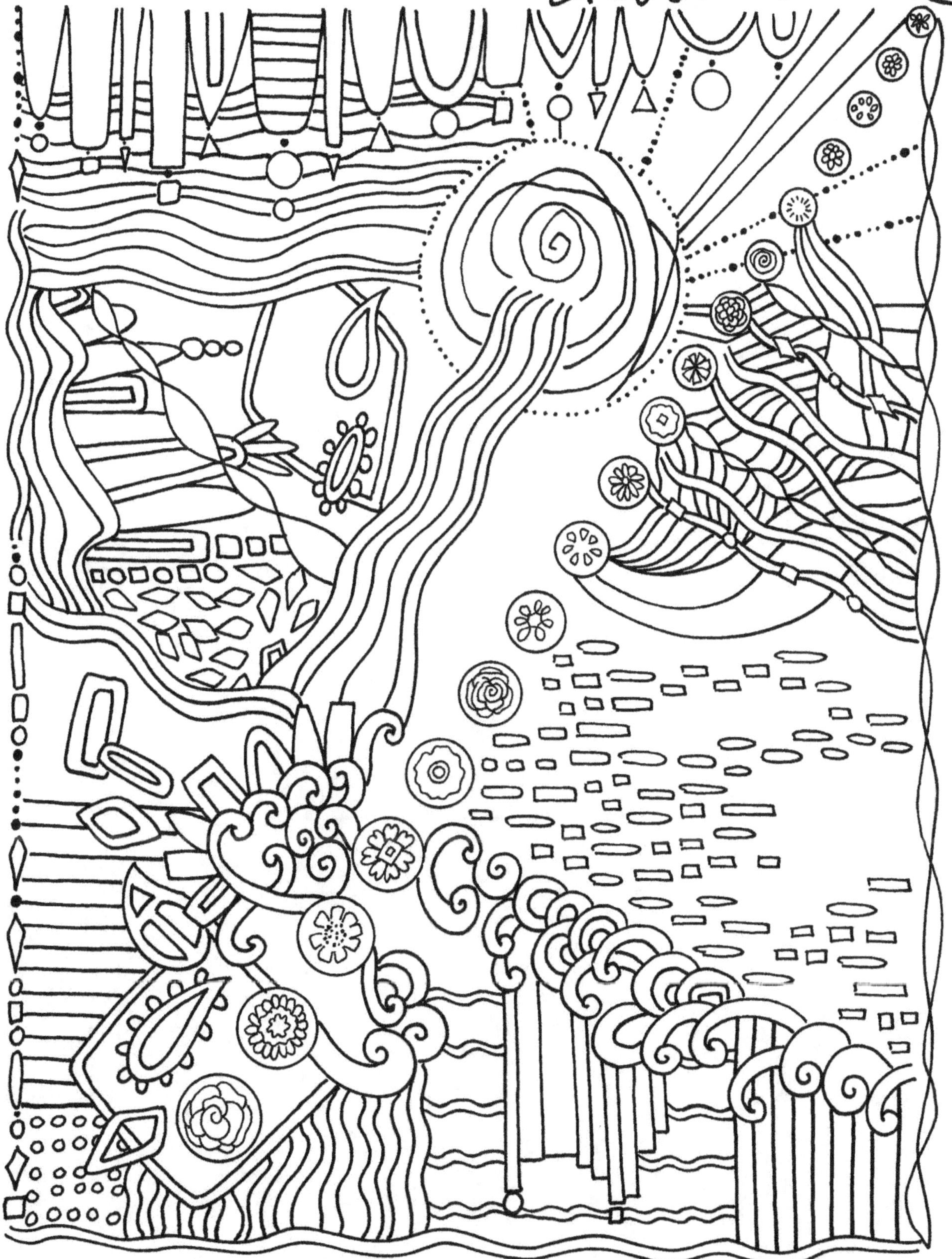

they are ADDICTED to escaping Reality

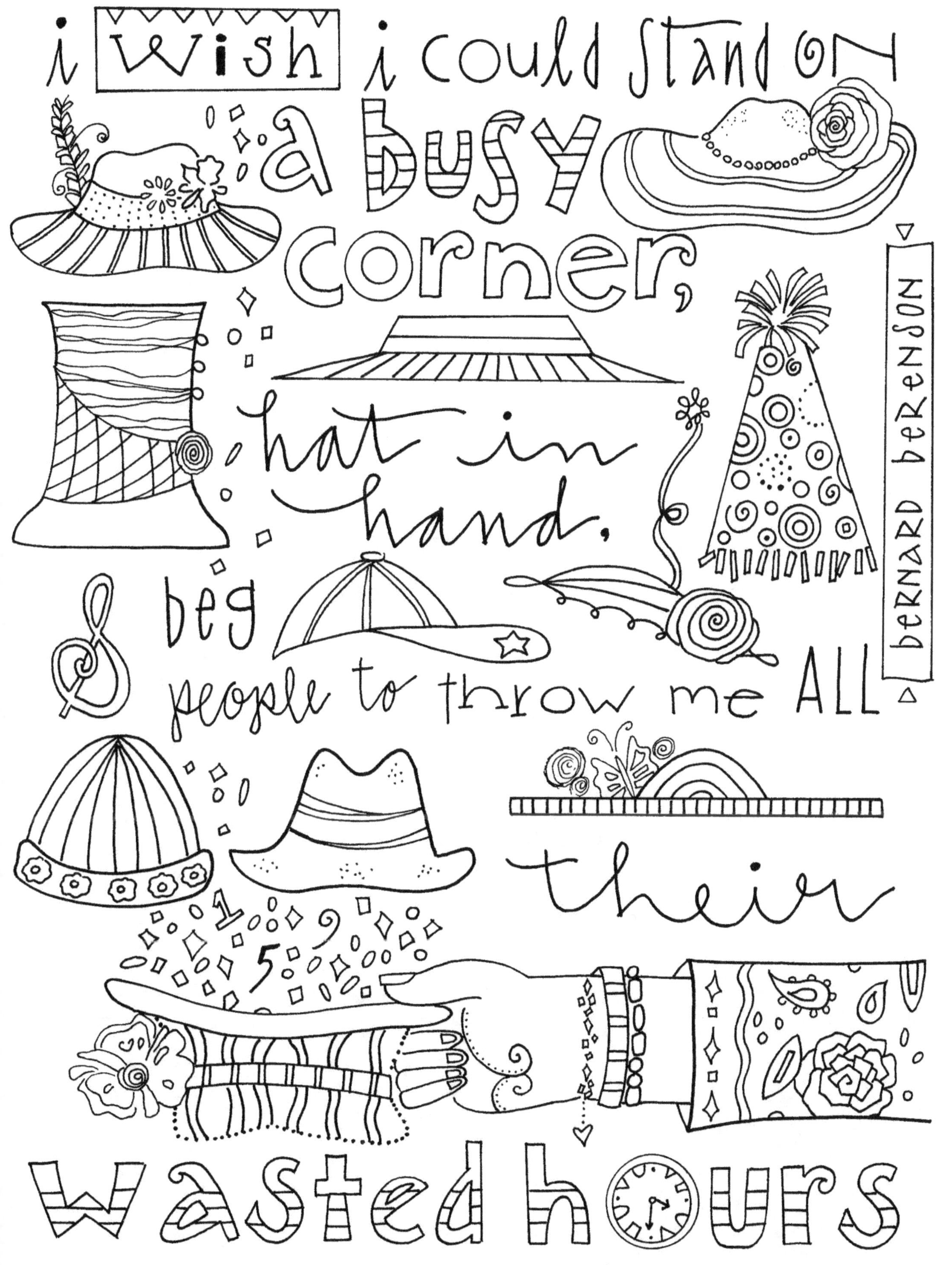

i wish i could stand on a busy corner, hat in hand, beg people to throw me ALL their wasted hours
BERNARD BERENSON

that Something "Out there"
can instantly
instantly fill up
Addiction begins with the hope
truth check
THINGS
FEELINGS
EXPERIENCES
PEOPLE
the emptiness INSIDE. — Jean Killbourne

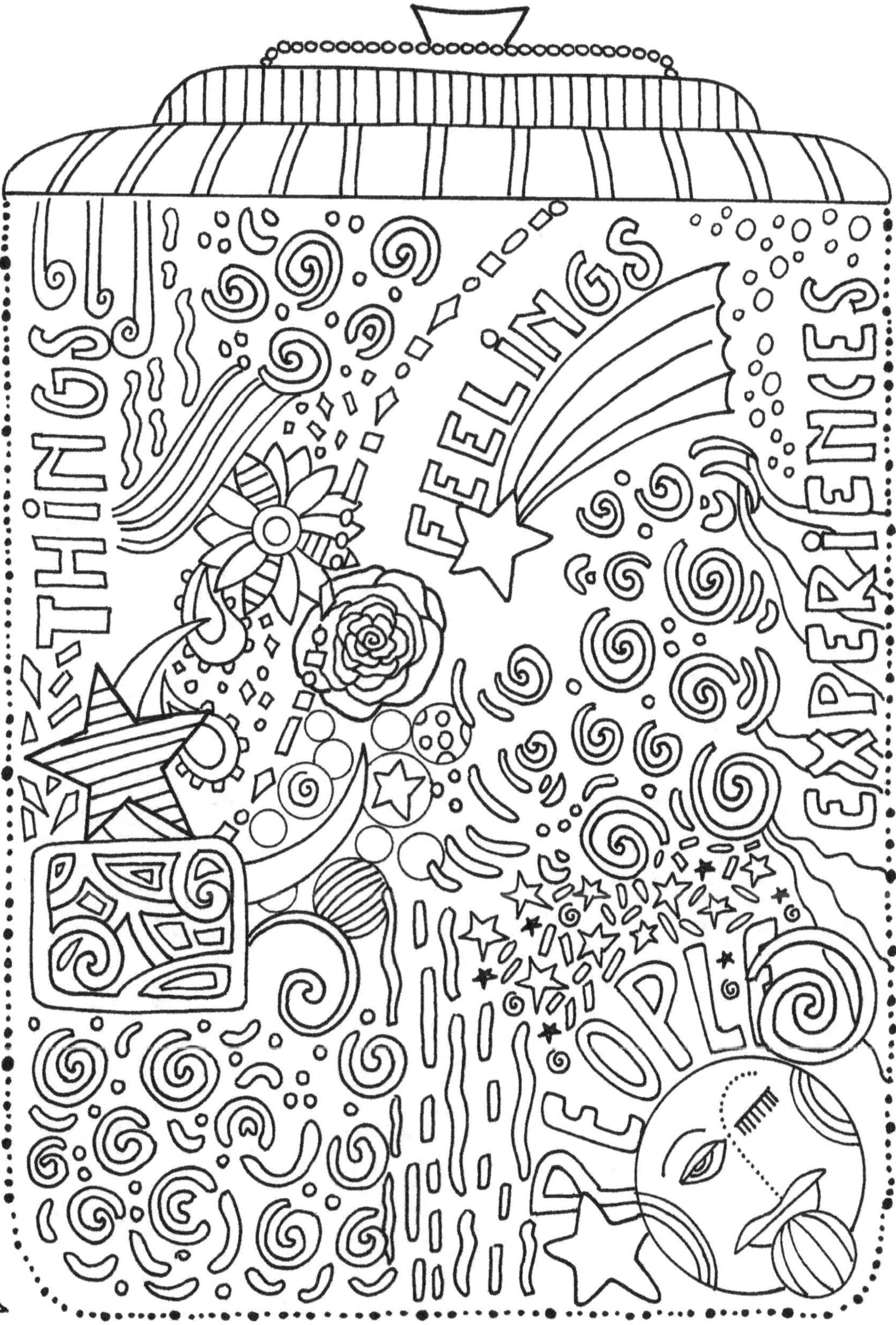

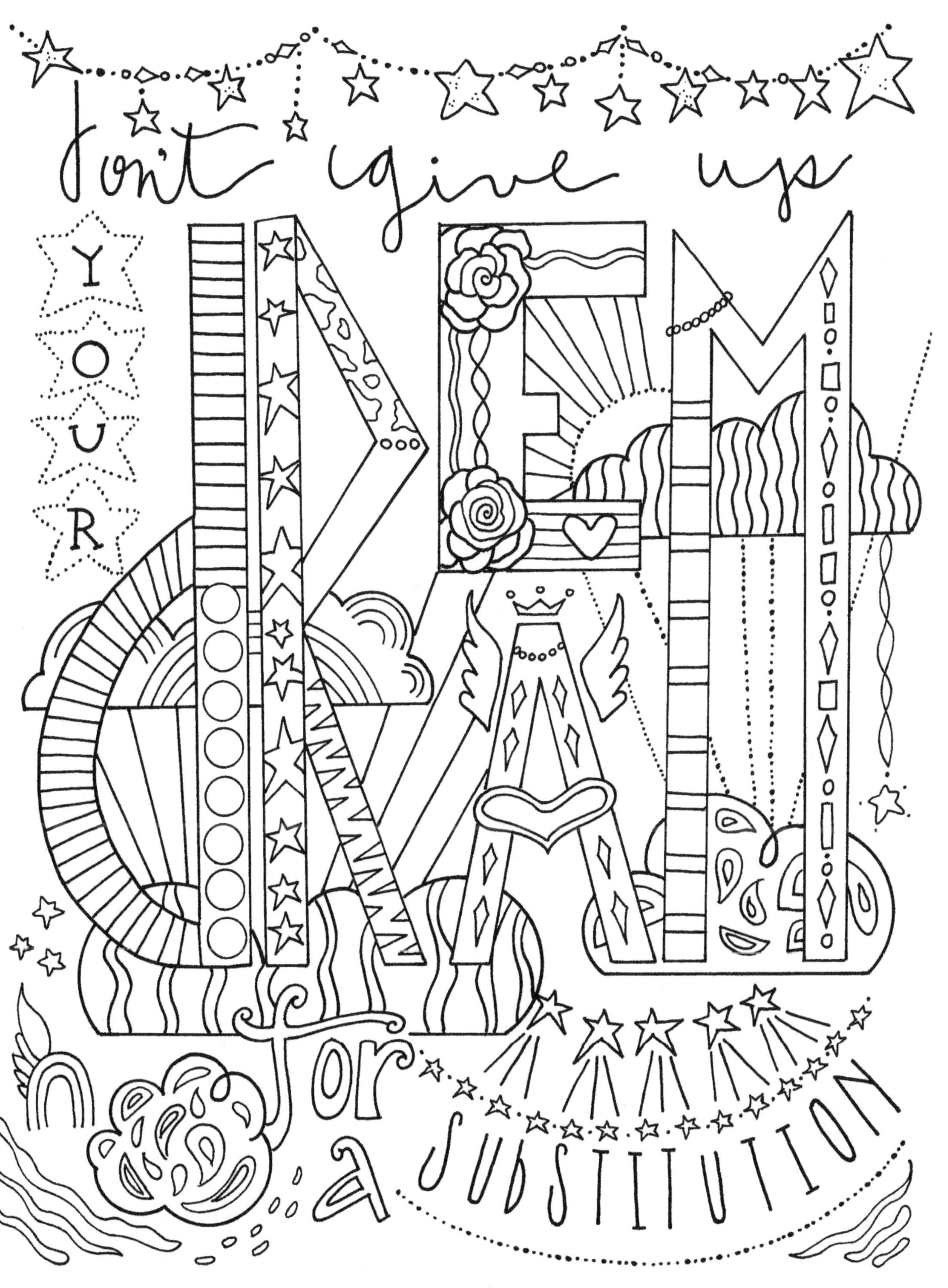

Don't give us
YOUR
DREAM
for a substitution

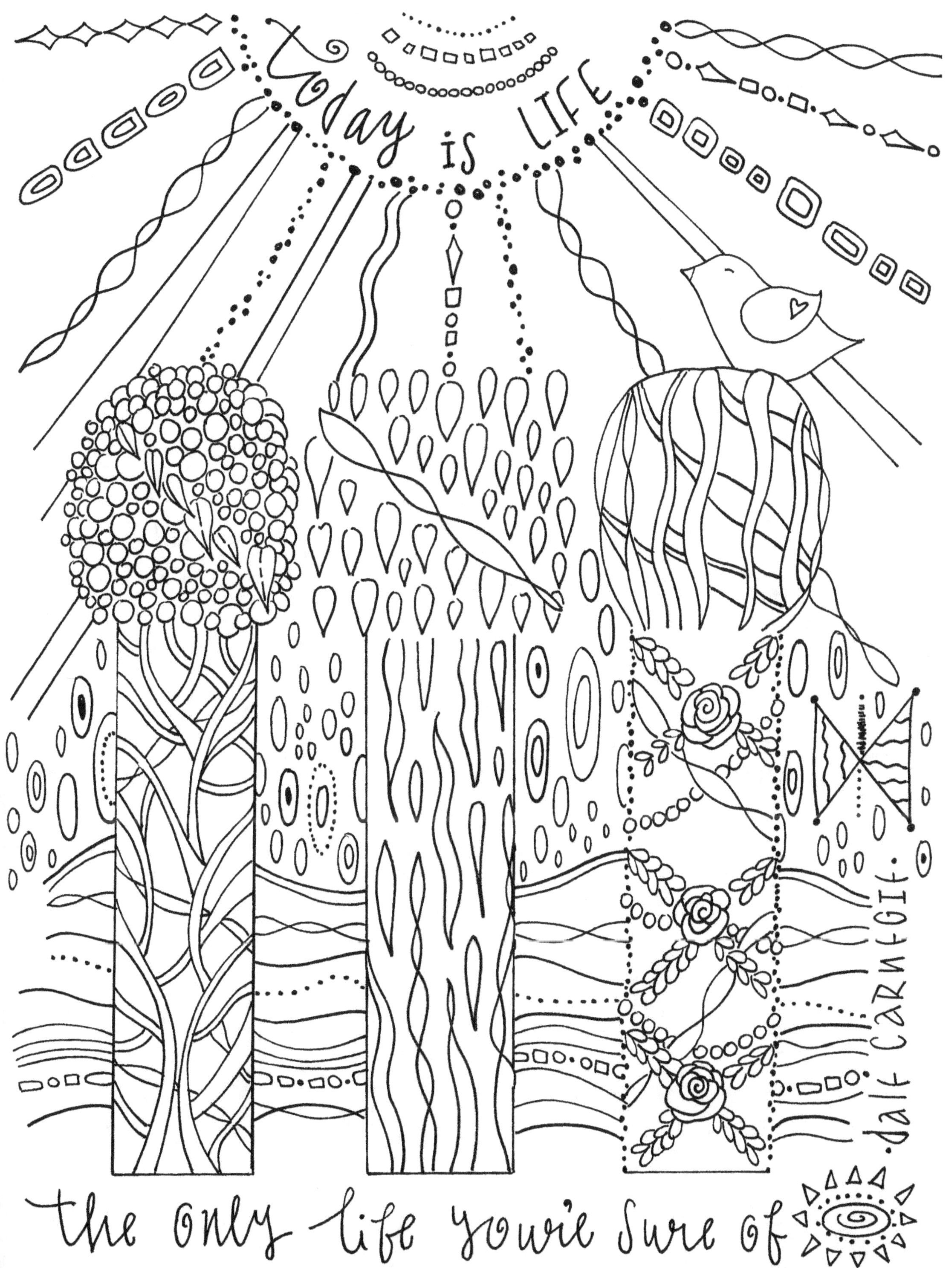

Today is LIFE
the only life you're sure of
-Dale Carnegie

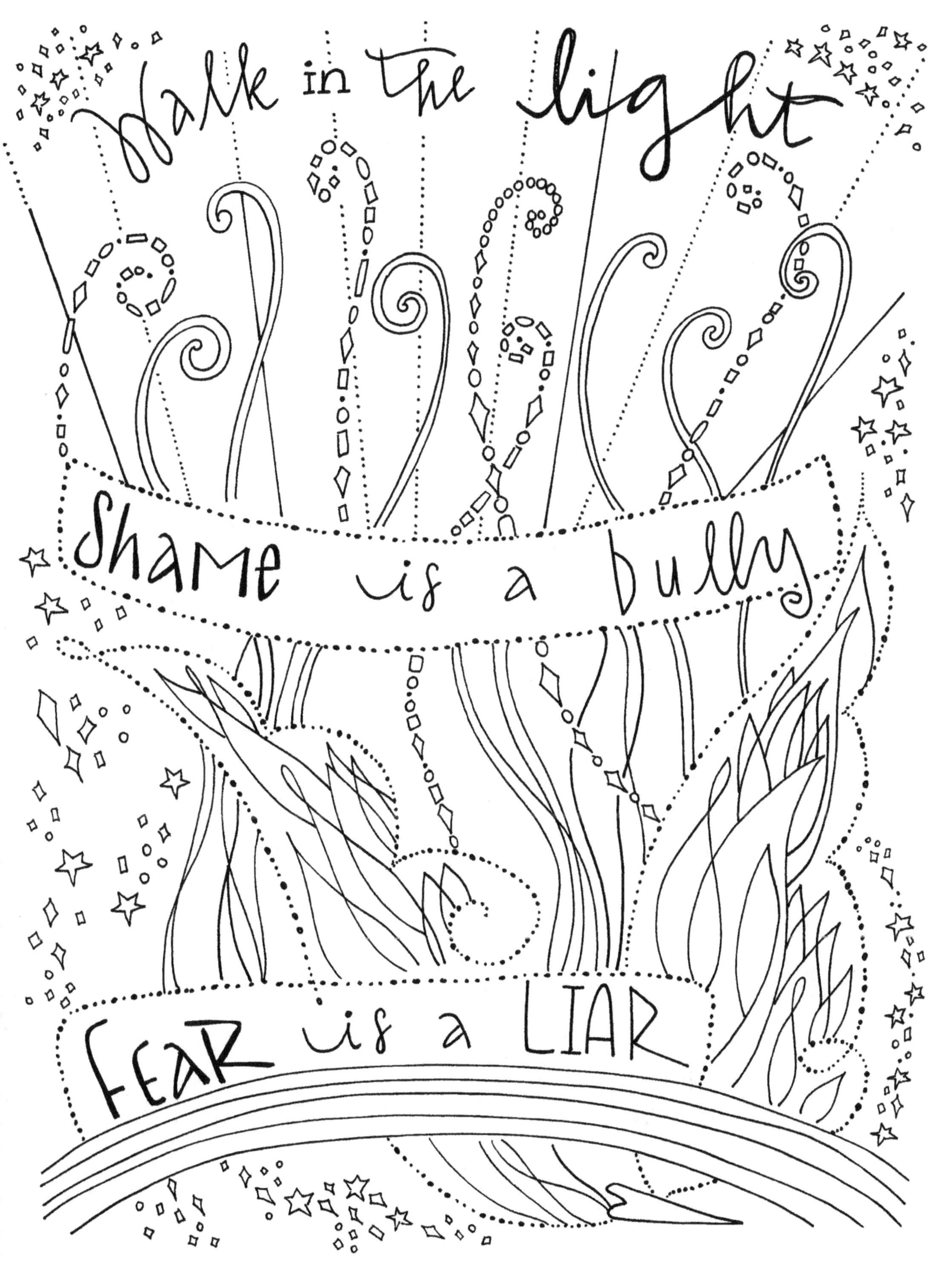

Walk in the light
Shame is a bully
FEAR is a LIAR

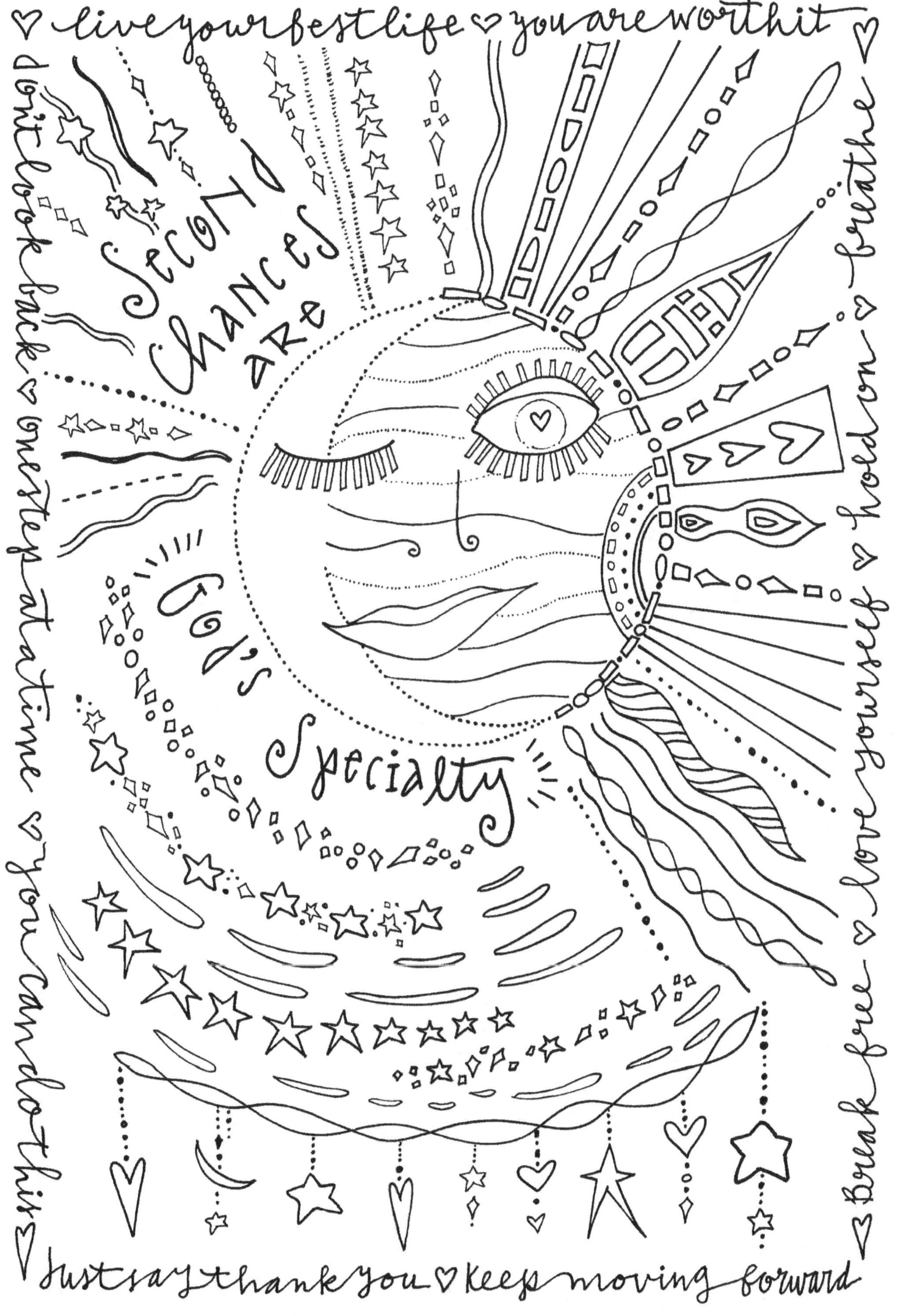

live your best life ♡ you are worth it
don't look back ♡ one step at a time ♡ you can do this
Second Chances are
God's Specialty
breathe ♡ hold on ♡ love yourself ♡ Break free
Just say thank you ♡ keep moving forward

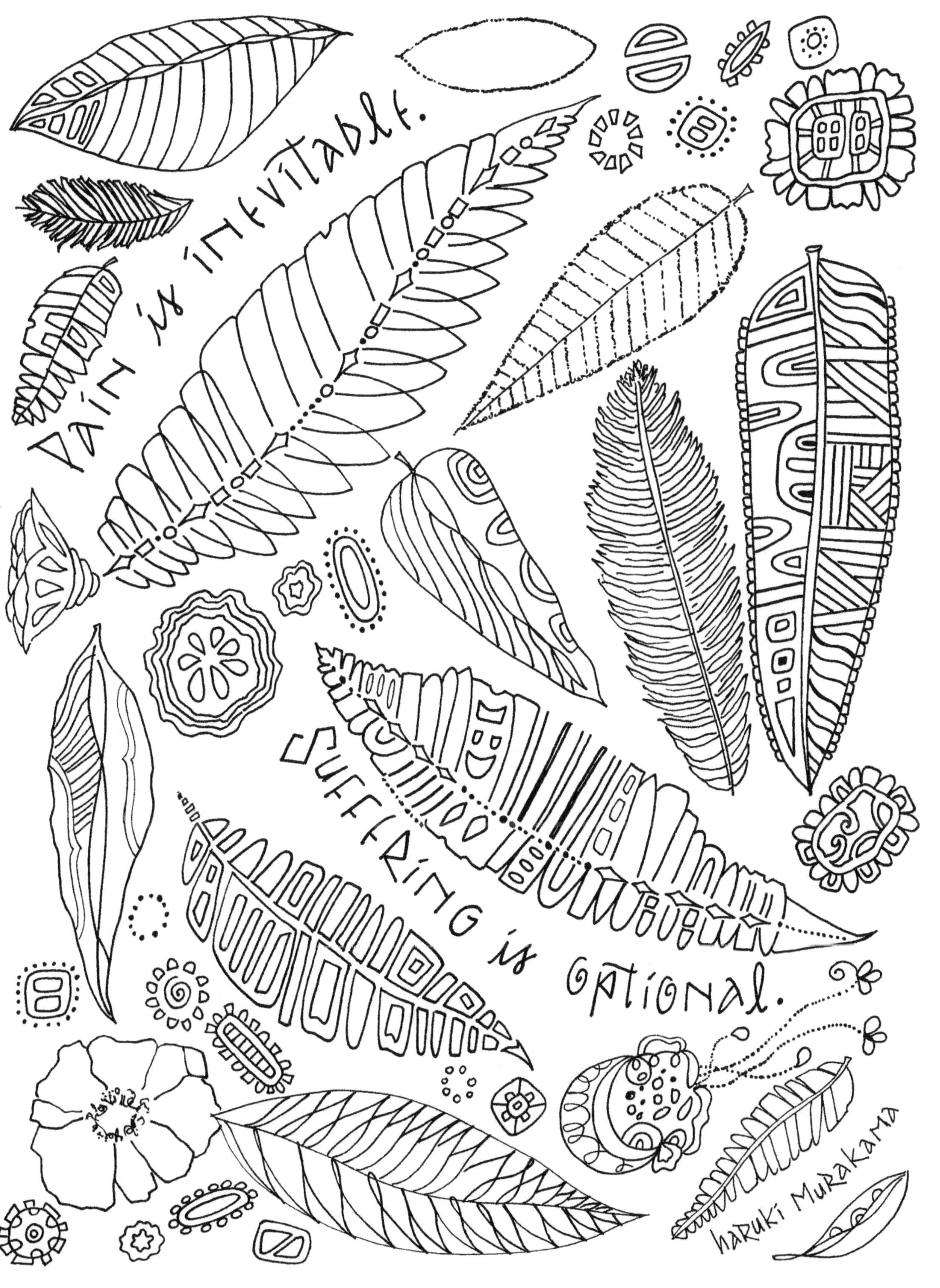

Pain is inevitable.
Suffering is optional.
Haruki Murakami

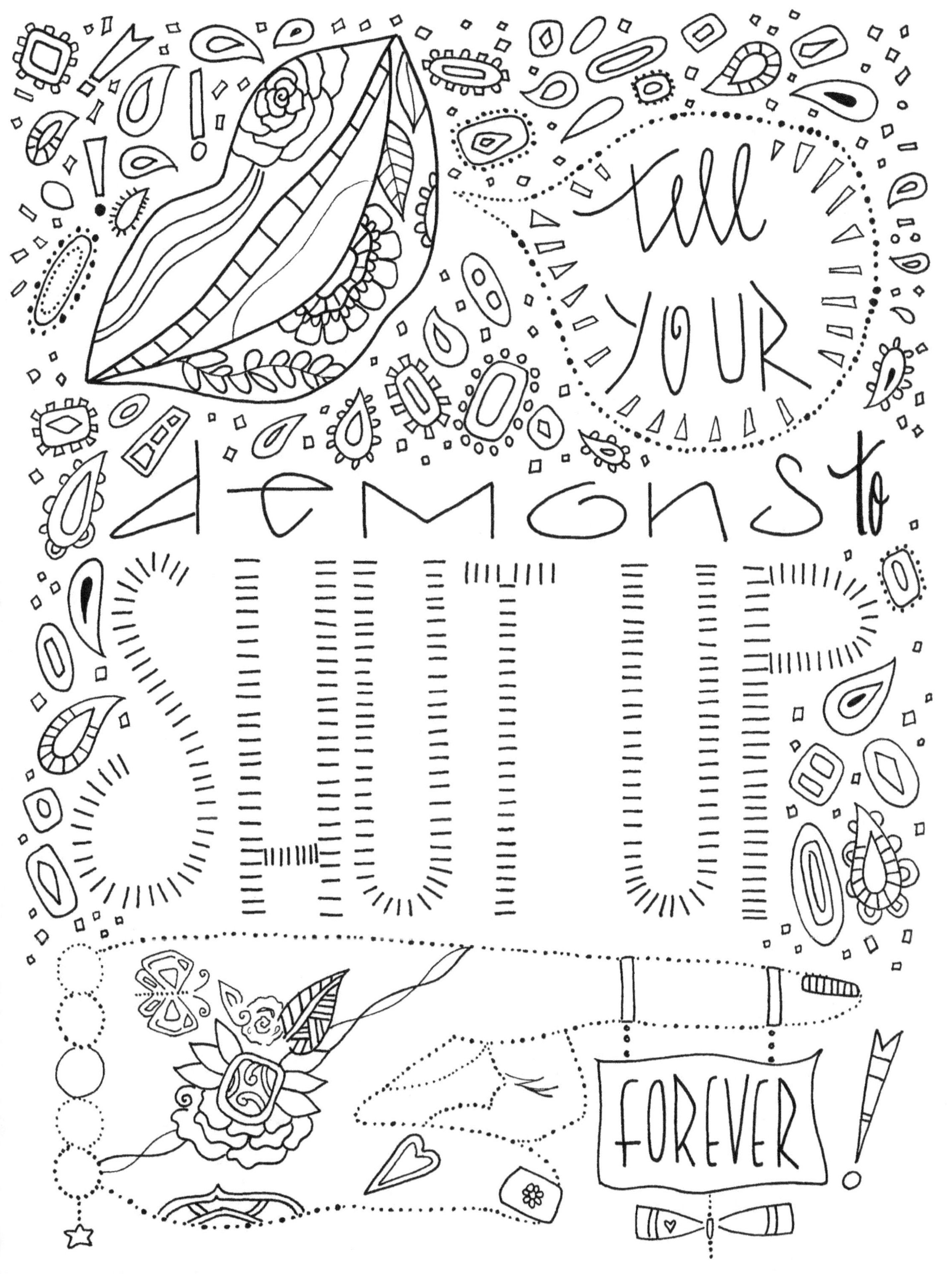

tell your
demons to
SHUT UP
FOREVER!

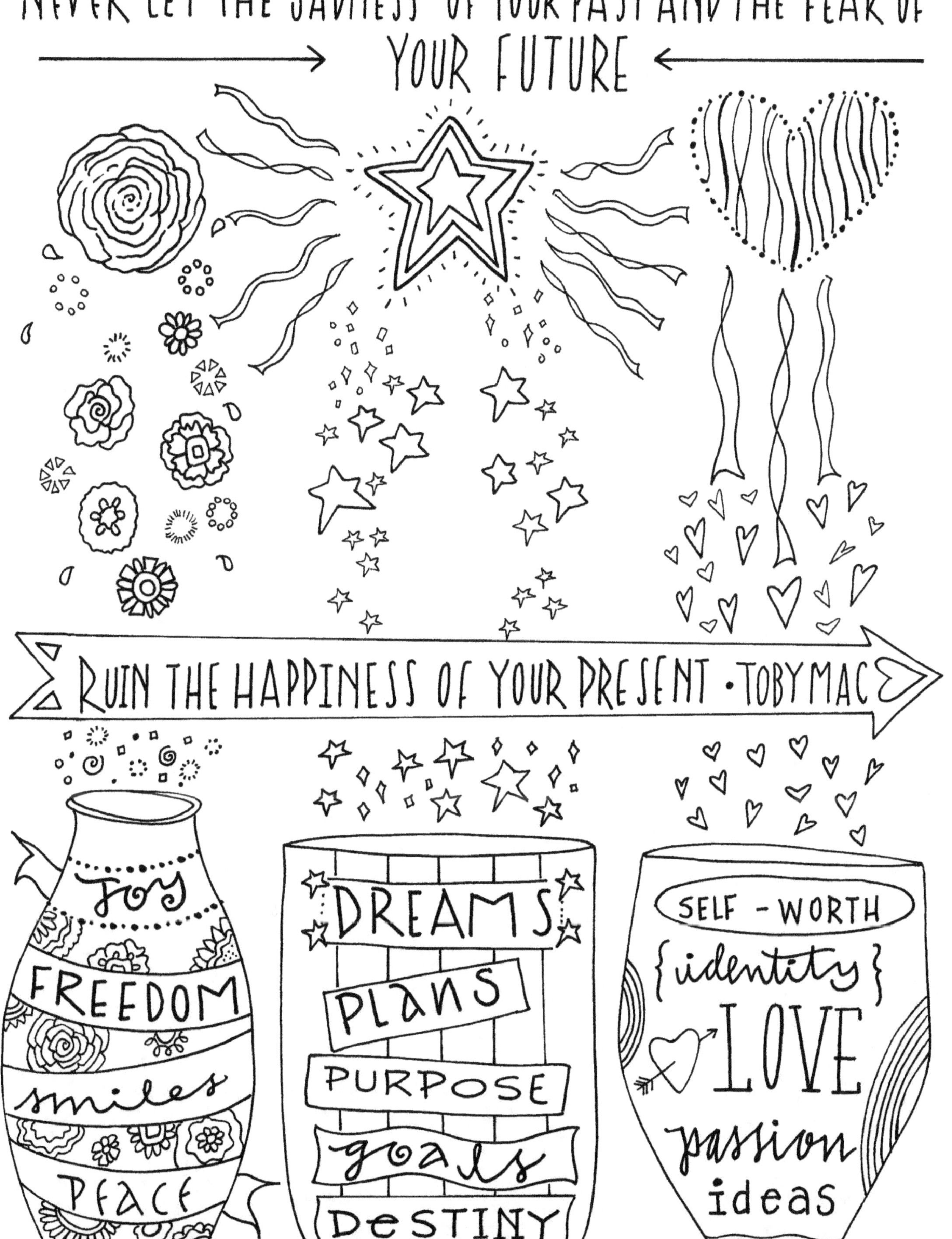

NEVER LET THE SADNESS OF YOUR PAST AND THE FEAR OF YOUR FUTURE
RUIN THE HAPPINESS OF YOUR PRESENT • TOBYMAC
Joy
FREEDOM
smiles
PEACE
DREAMS
PLANS
PURPOSE
goals
DESTINY
SELF - WORTH
{identity}
LOVE
passion
ideas

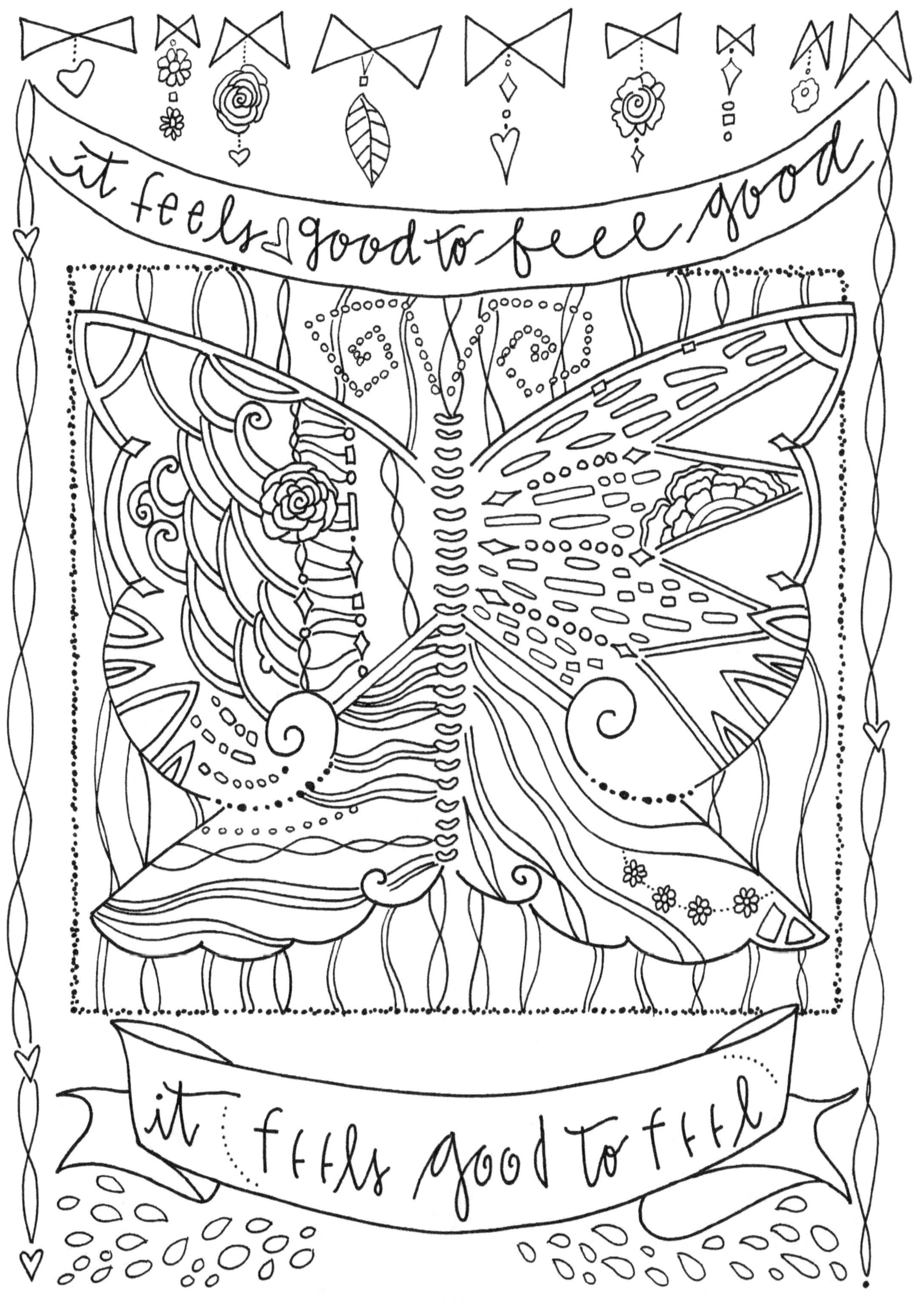

it feels good to feel good
it feels good to feel!

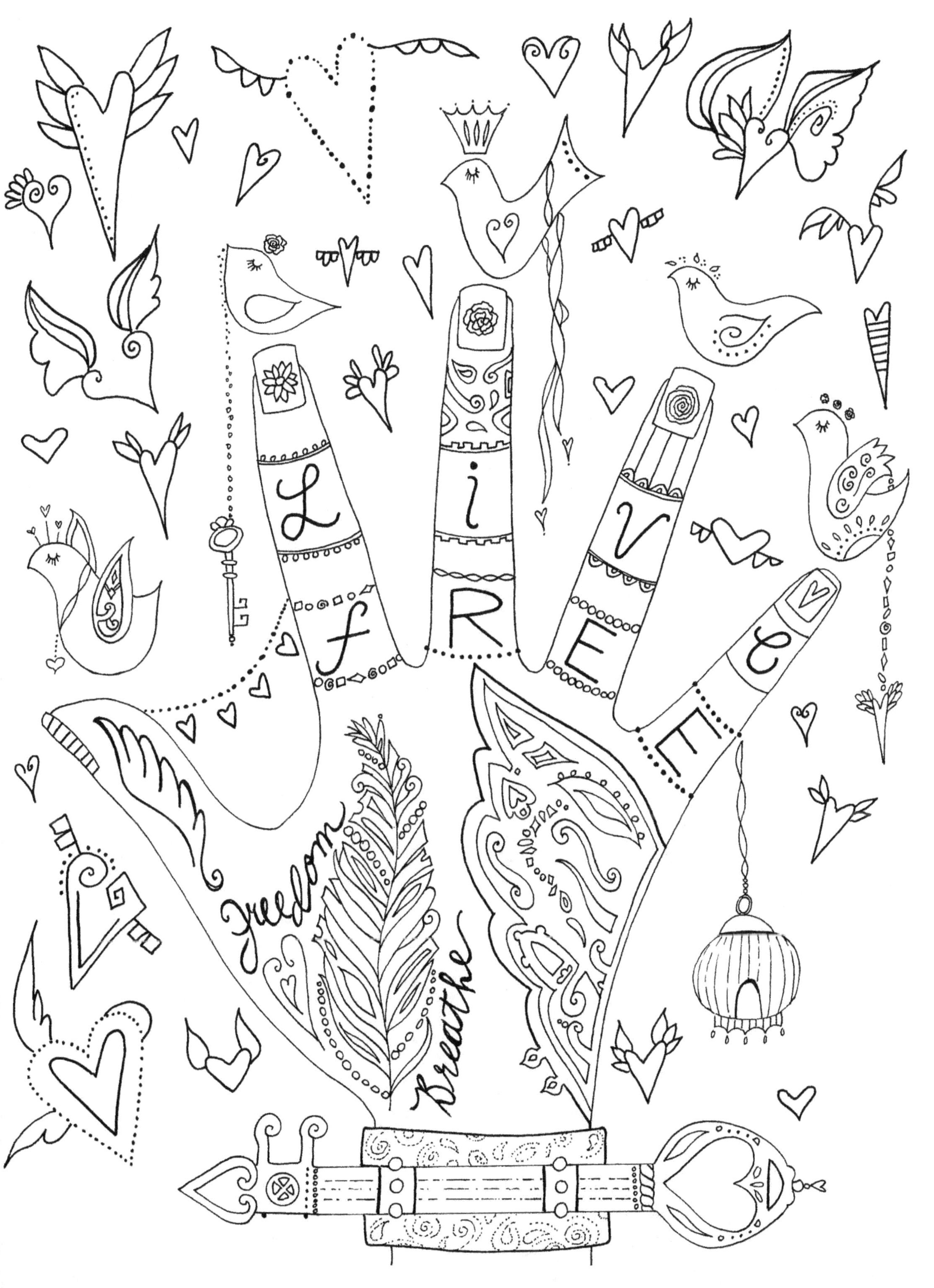

Live free
Freedom
breathe

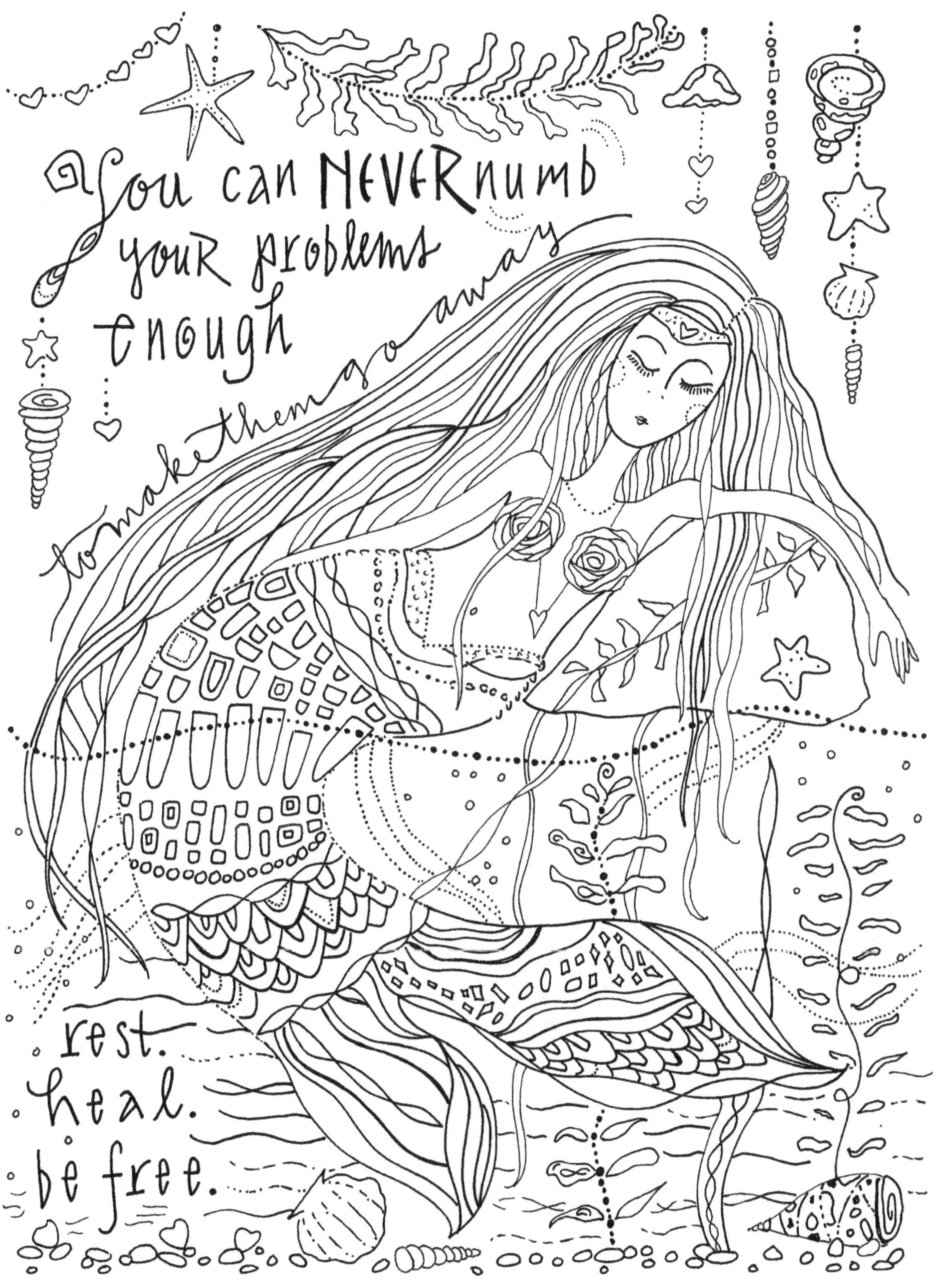
You can NEVER numb your problems enough
to make them go away
rest.
heal.
be free.

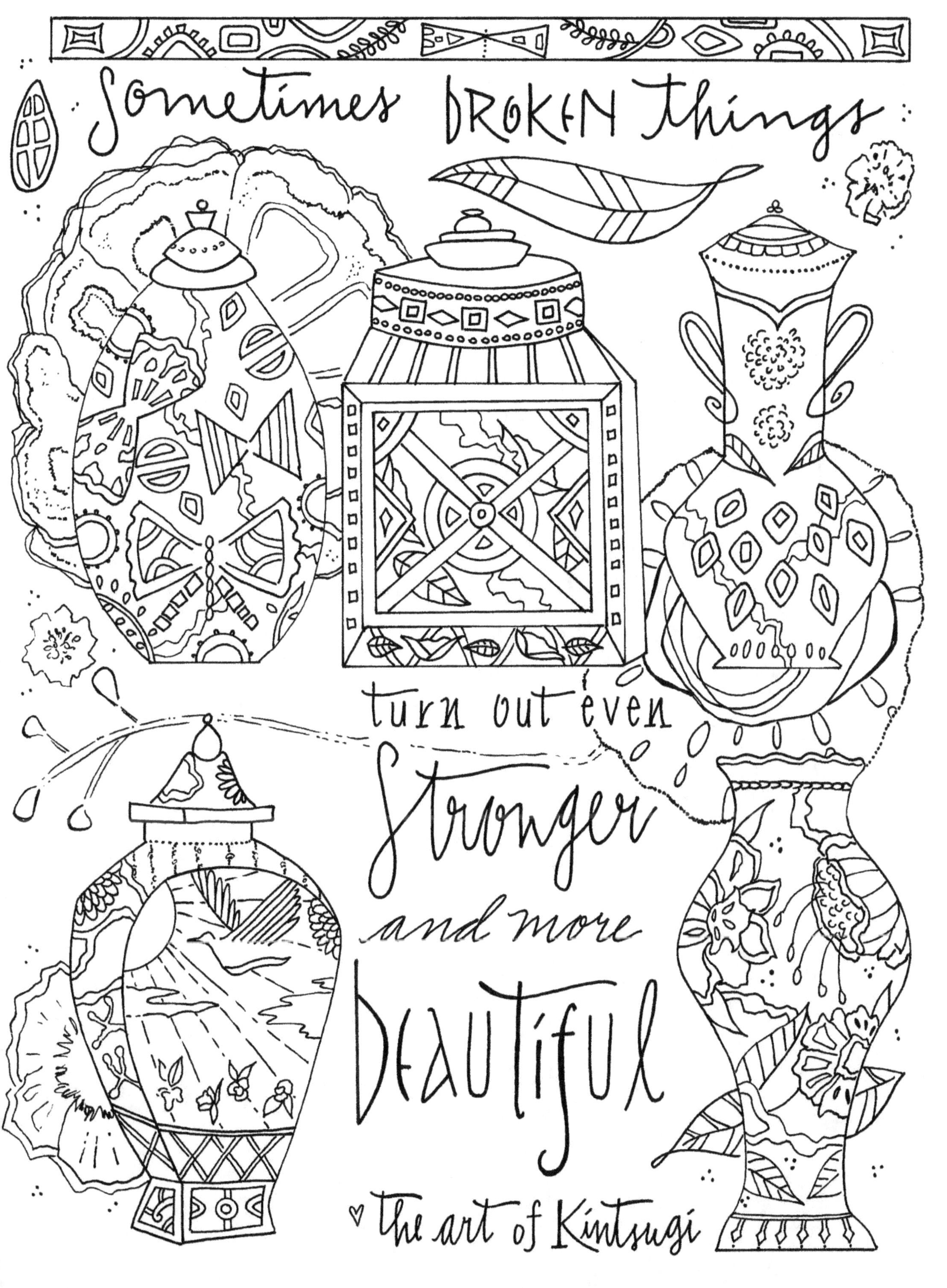

Sometimes BROKEN things
turn out even
Stronger
and more
beautiful
♥ the art of Kintsugi

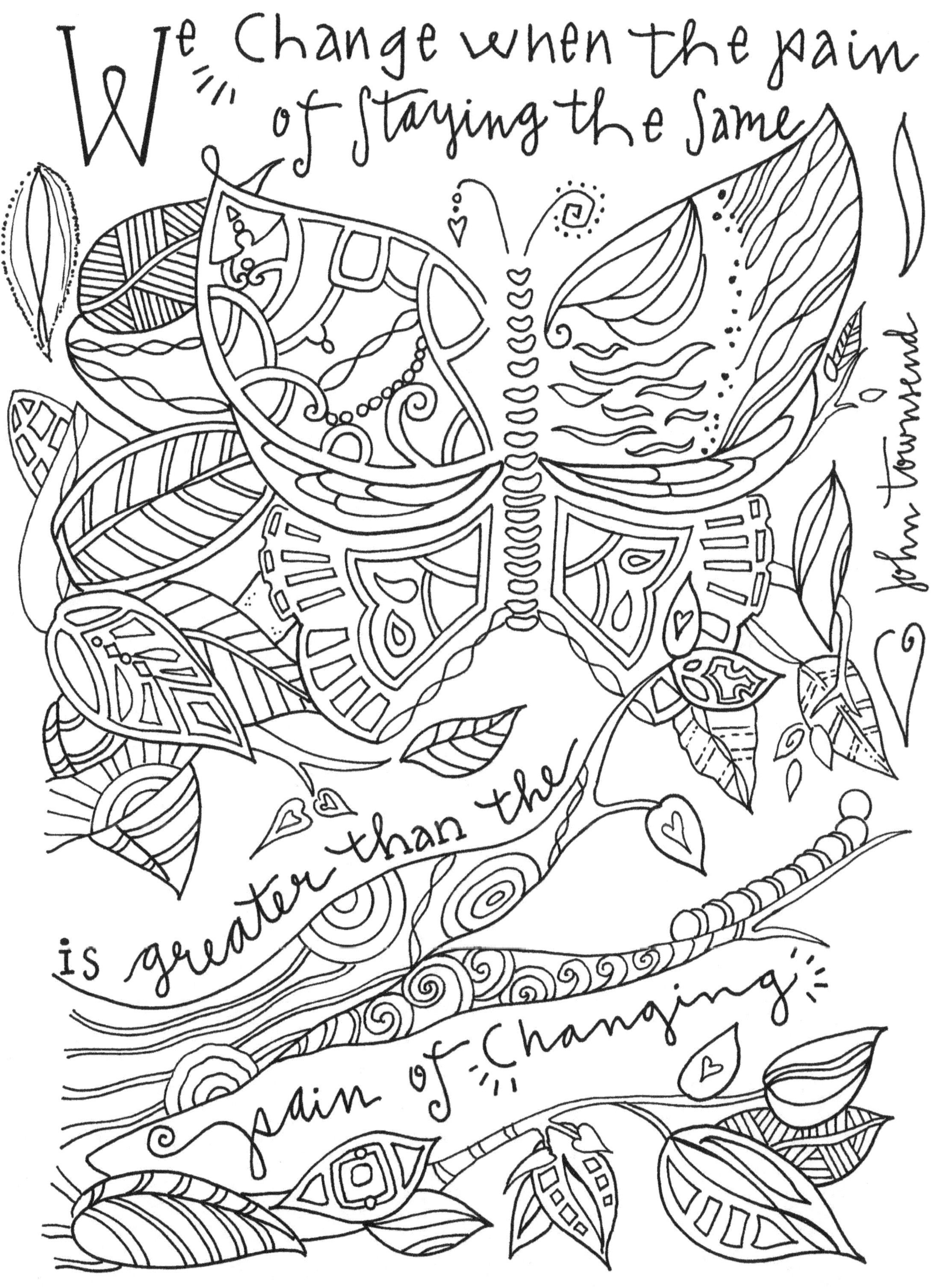

We change when the pain of staying the same
is greater than the
pain of changing
John Townsend

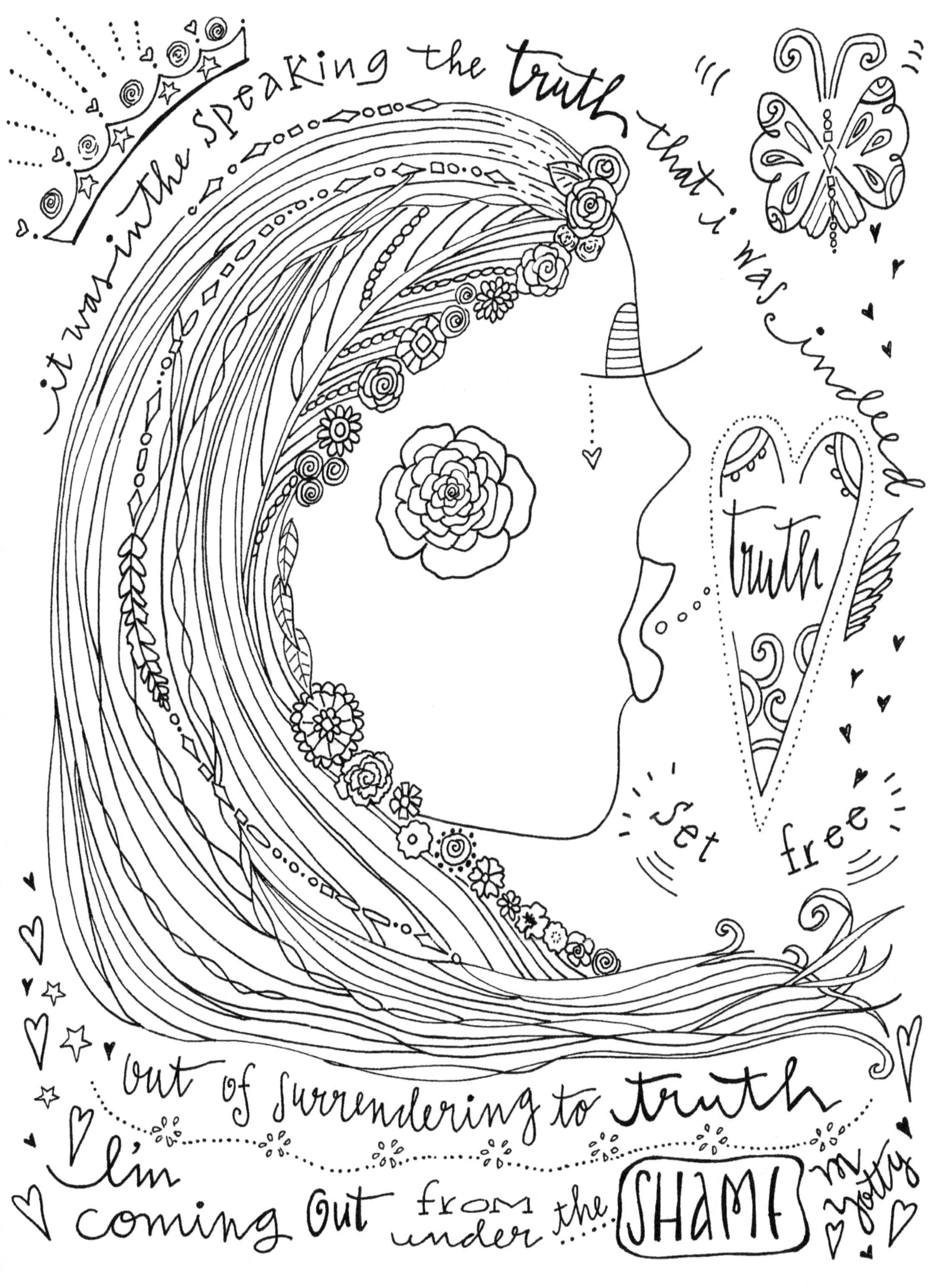

it was in the speaking the truth that i was indeed
truth
set free
out of surrendering to truth
I'm coming out from under the SHAME
m.yotty

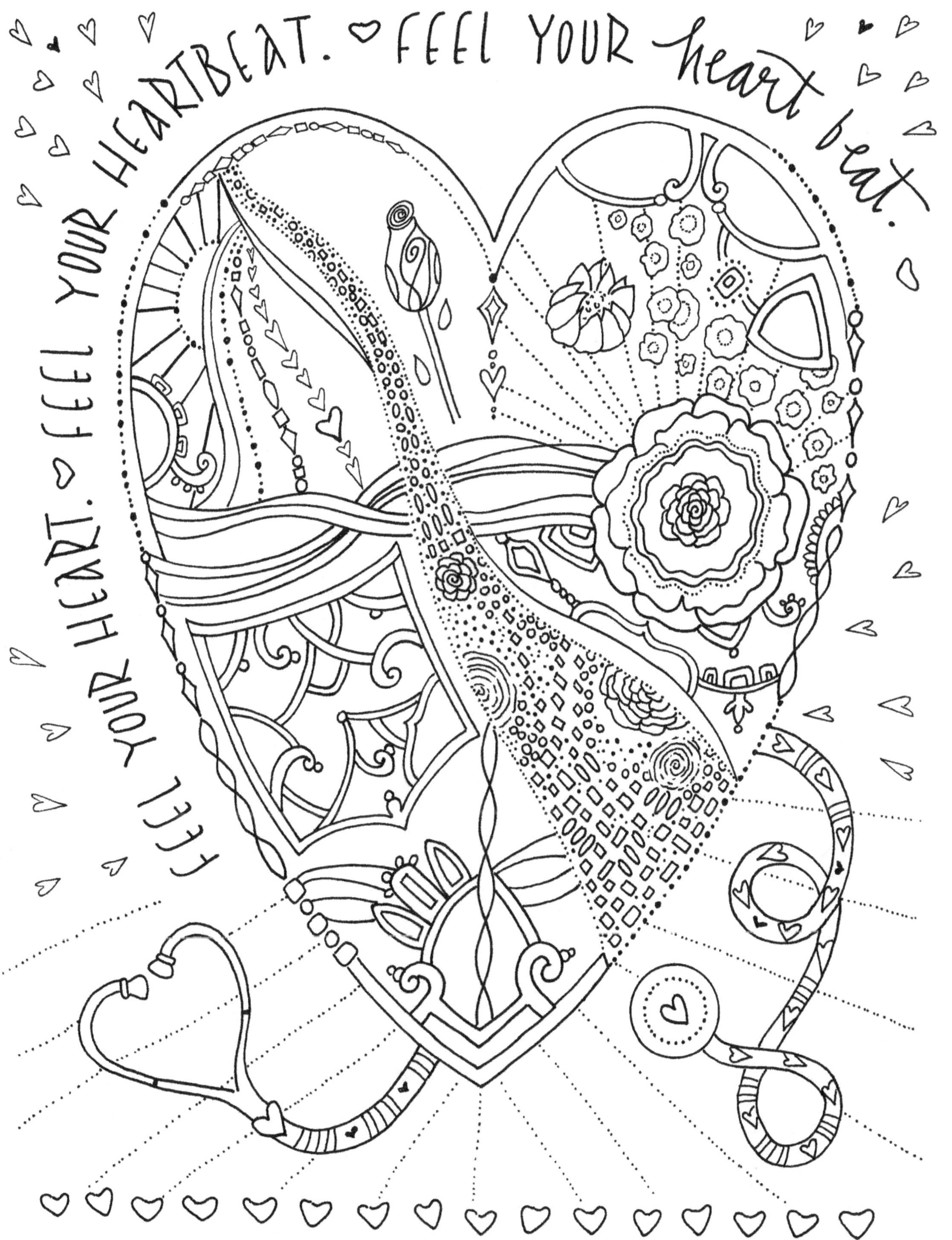
FEEL YOUR HEARTBEAT. FEEL YOUR heart beat.
FEEL YOUR HEART.
FEEL YOUR HEART.

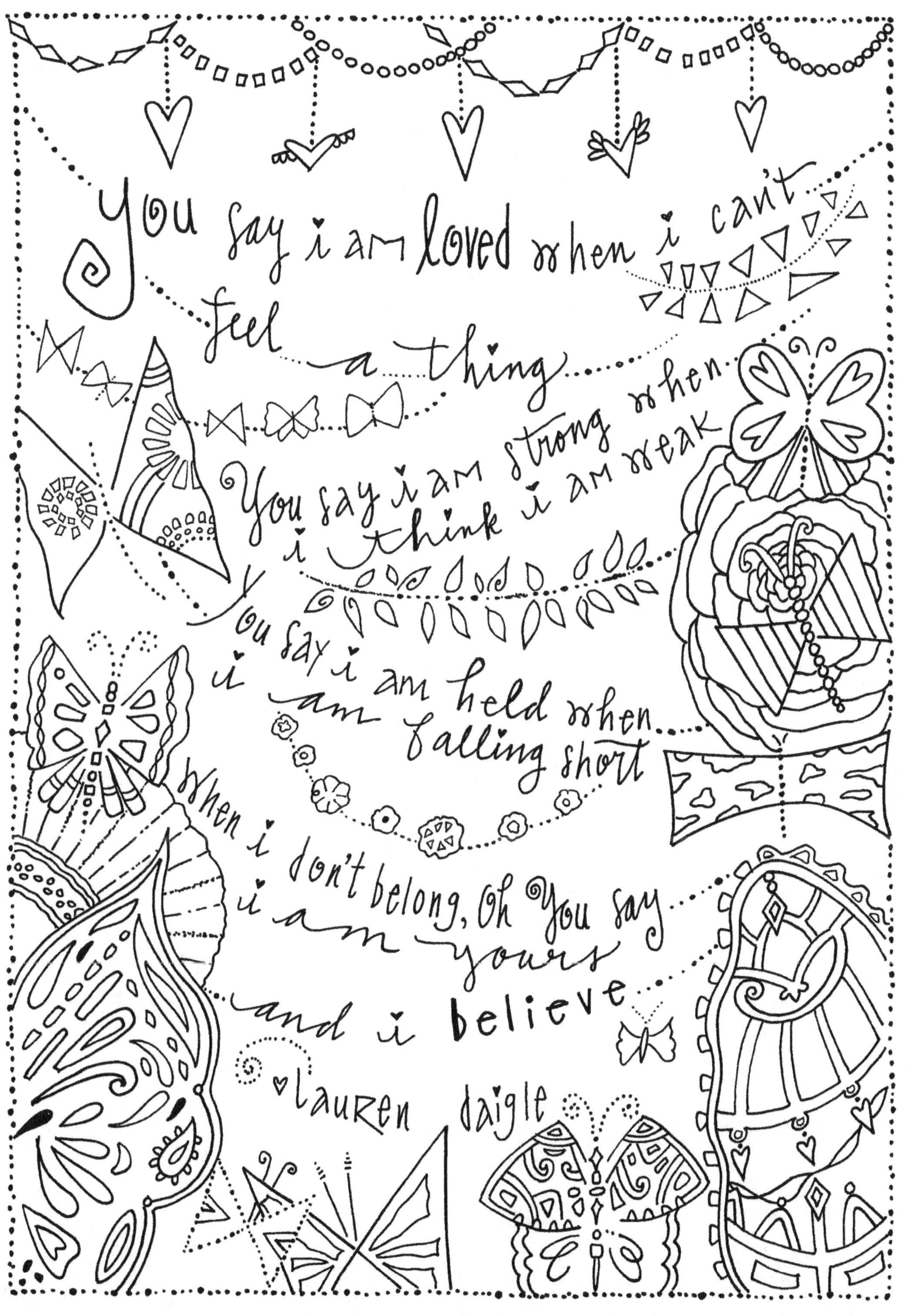

You say i am loved when i can't feel a thing
You say i am strong when i think i am weak
You say i am held when i am falling short
When i don't belong, Oh You say i am yours
and i believe
♥lauren daigle

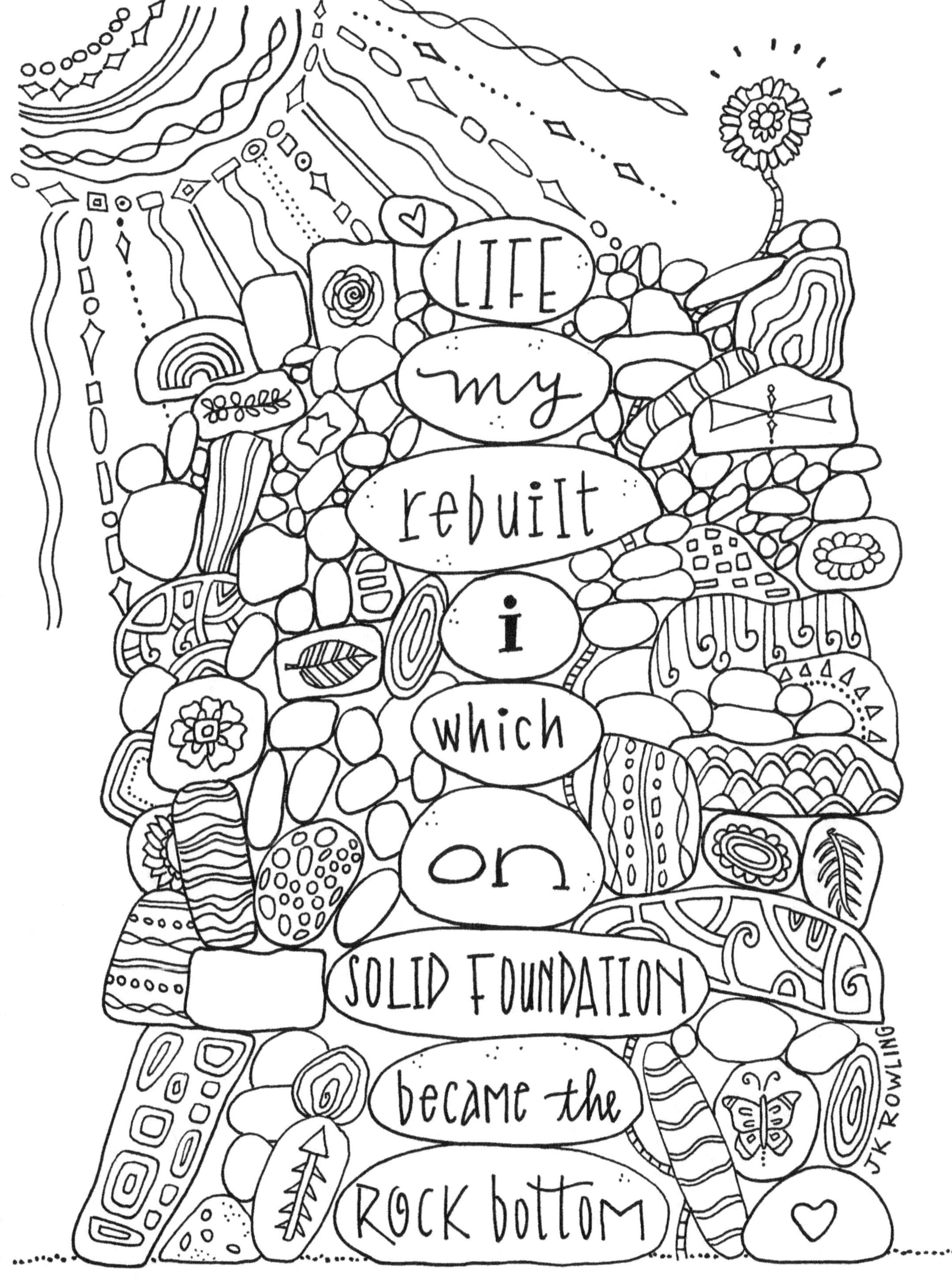

LIFE
my
rebuilt
i
which
on
SOLID FOUNDATION
became the
ROCK bottom
JK ROWLING

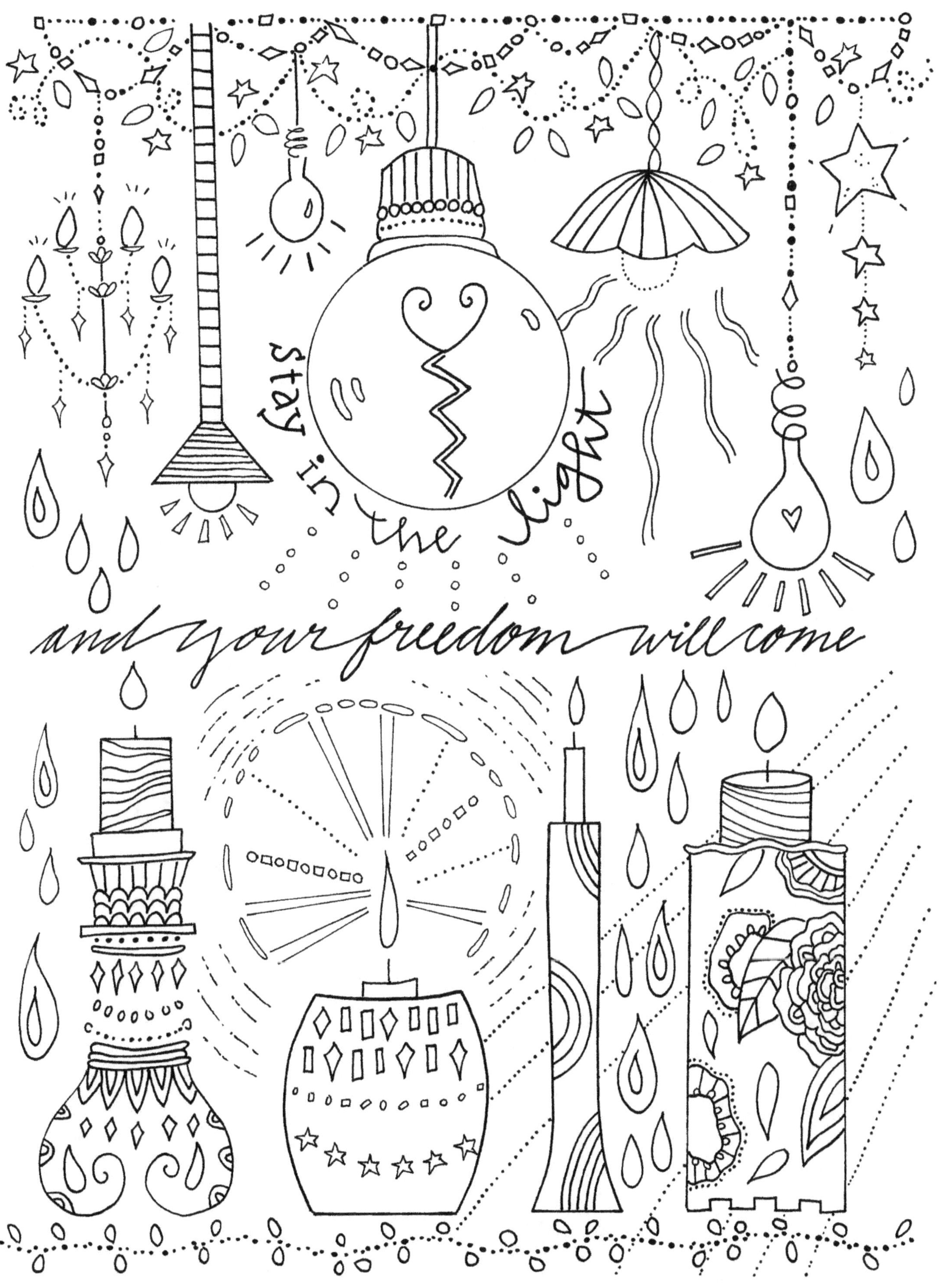

stay in the light
and your freedom will come

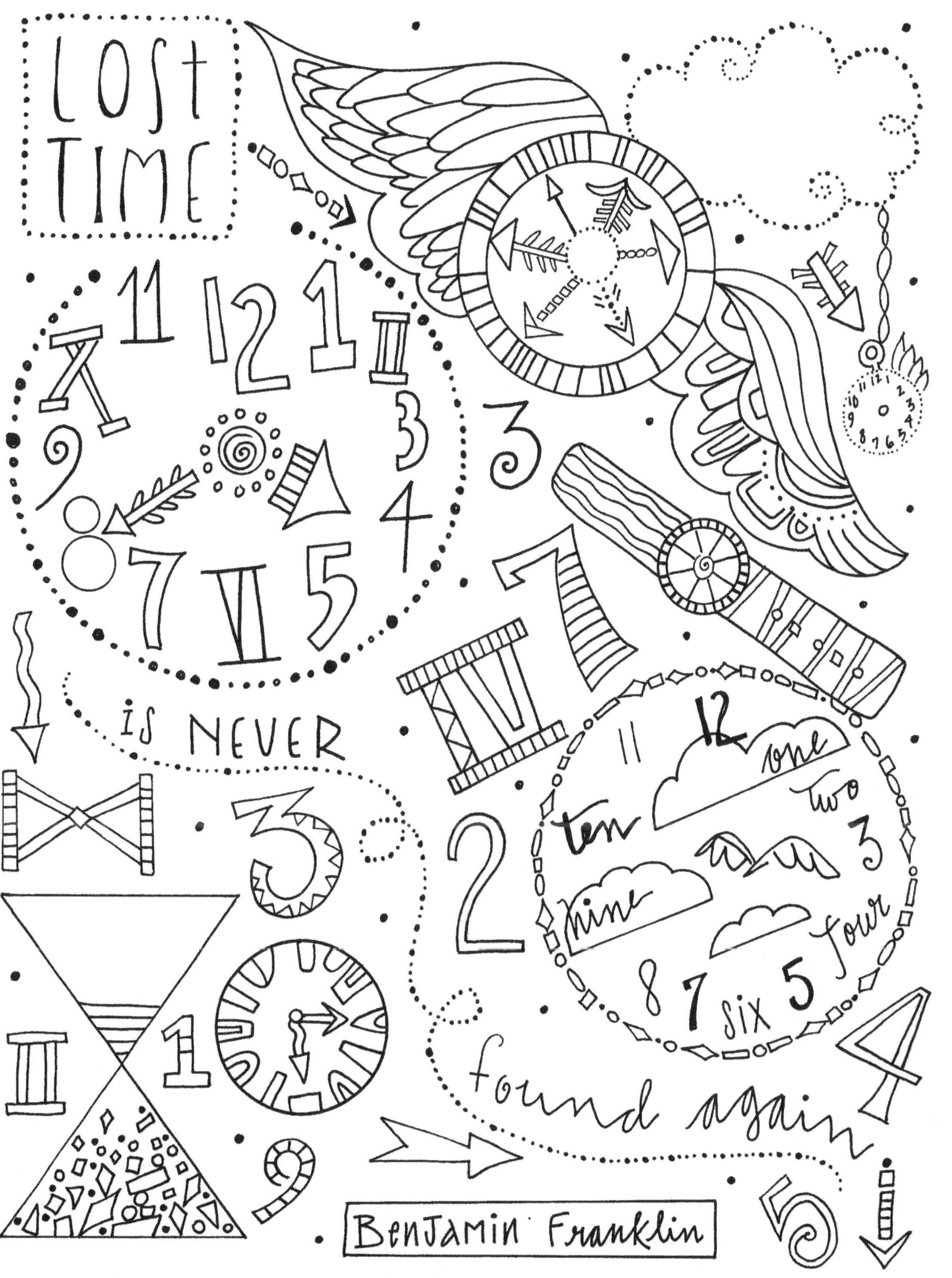

LOST TIME
is NEVER
found again
Benjamin Franklin

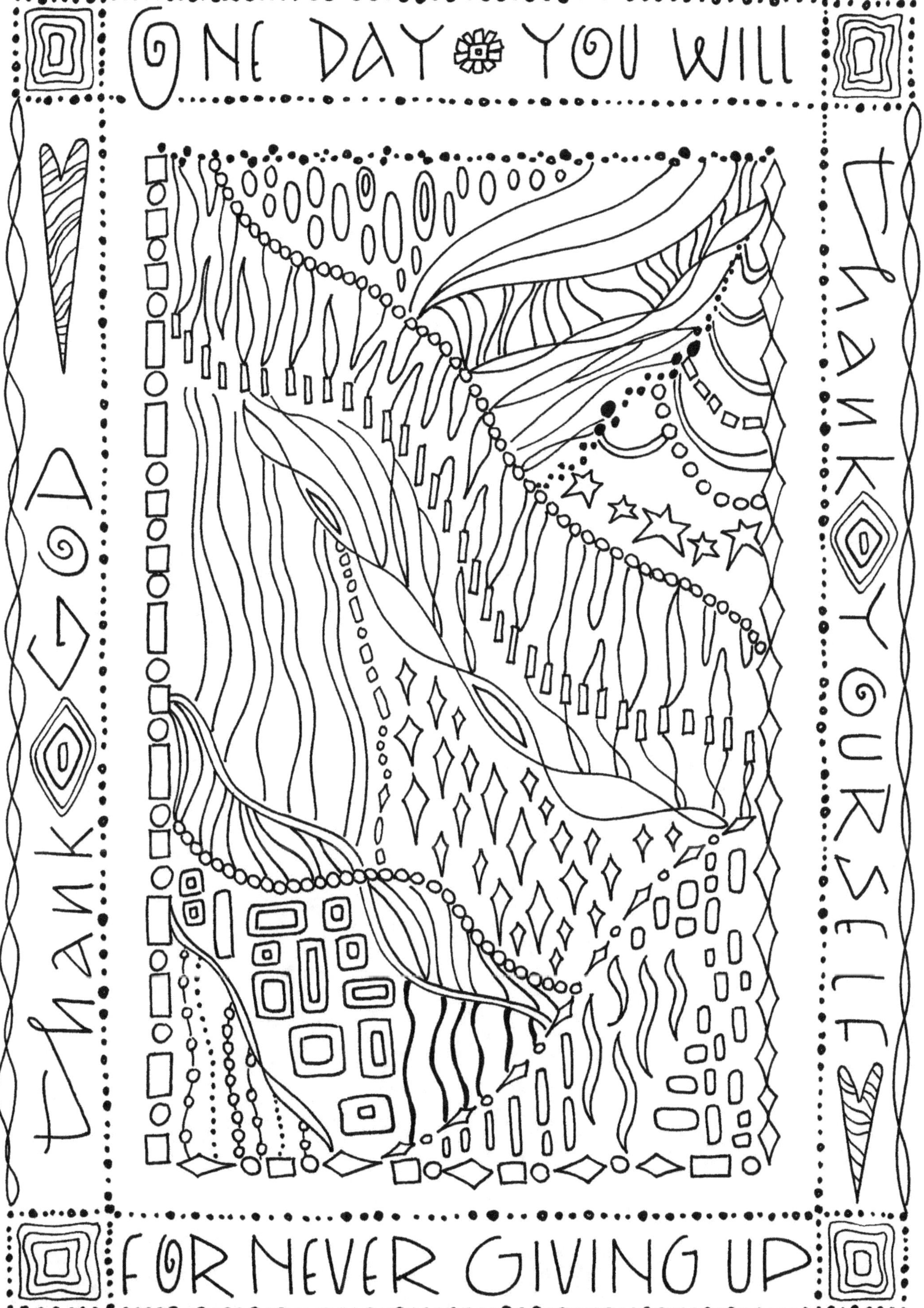

ONE DAY YOU WILL
THANK YOURSELF
FOR NEVER GIVING UP
THANK GOD

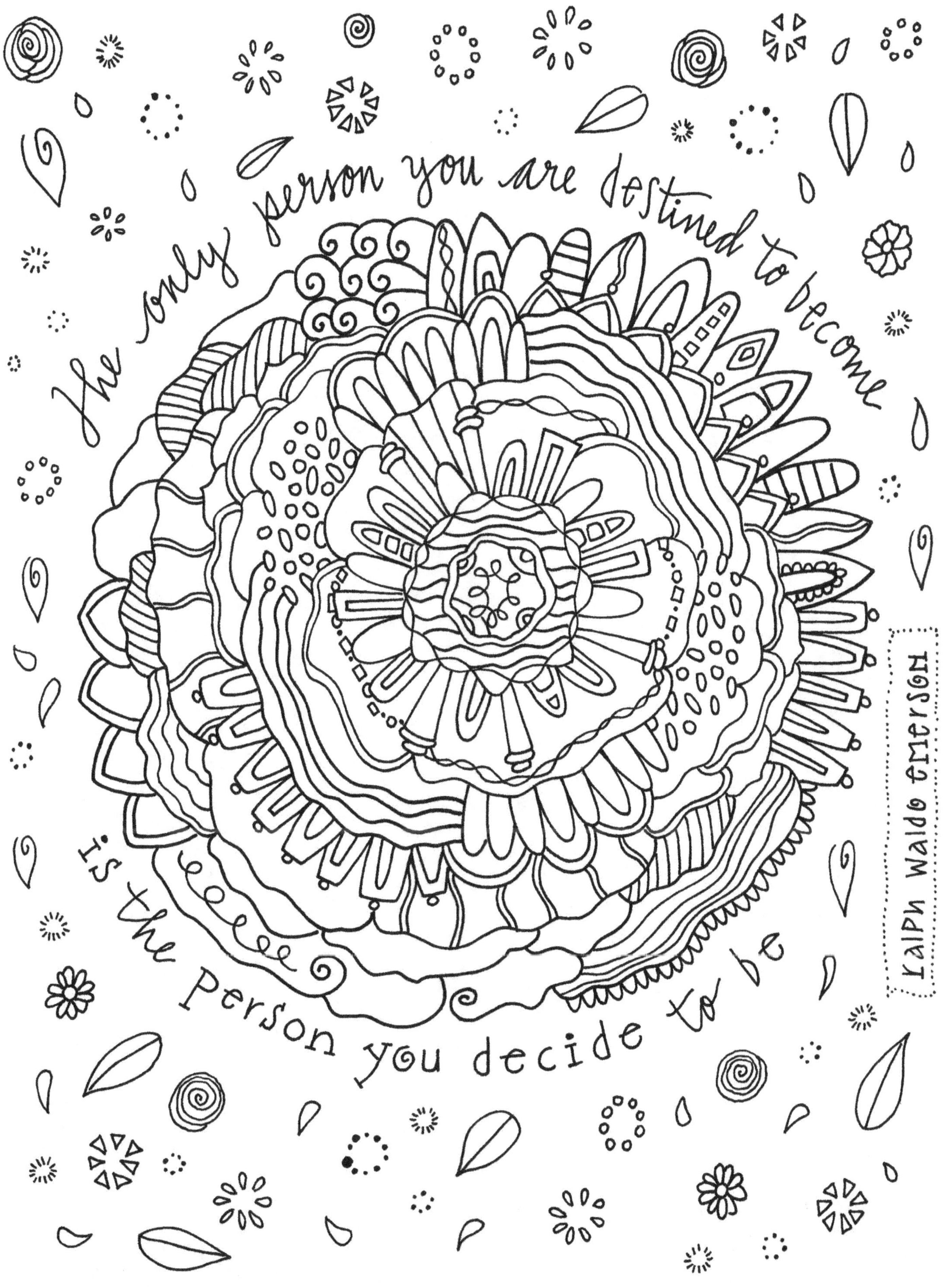
The only person you are destined to become
is the person you decide to be
Ralph Waldo Emerson

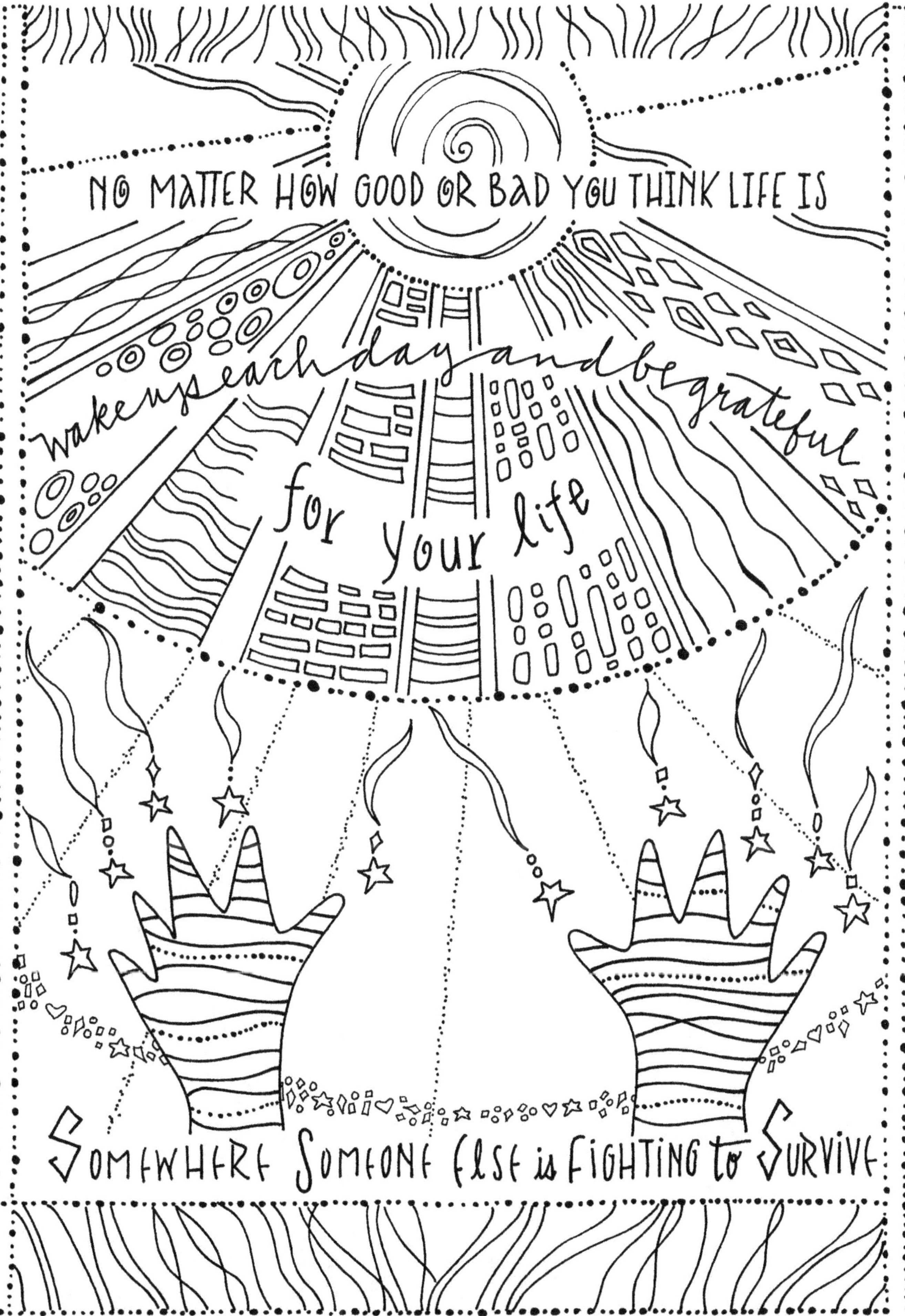

NO MATTER HOW GOOD OR BAD YOU THINK LIFE IS
wake up each day and be grateful
for your life
SOMEWHERE SOMEONE ELSE is FIGHTING to SURVIVE

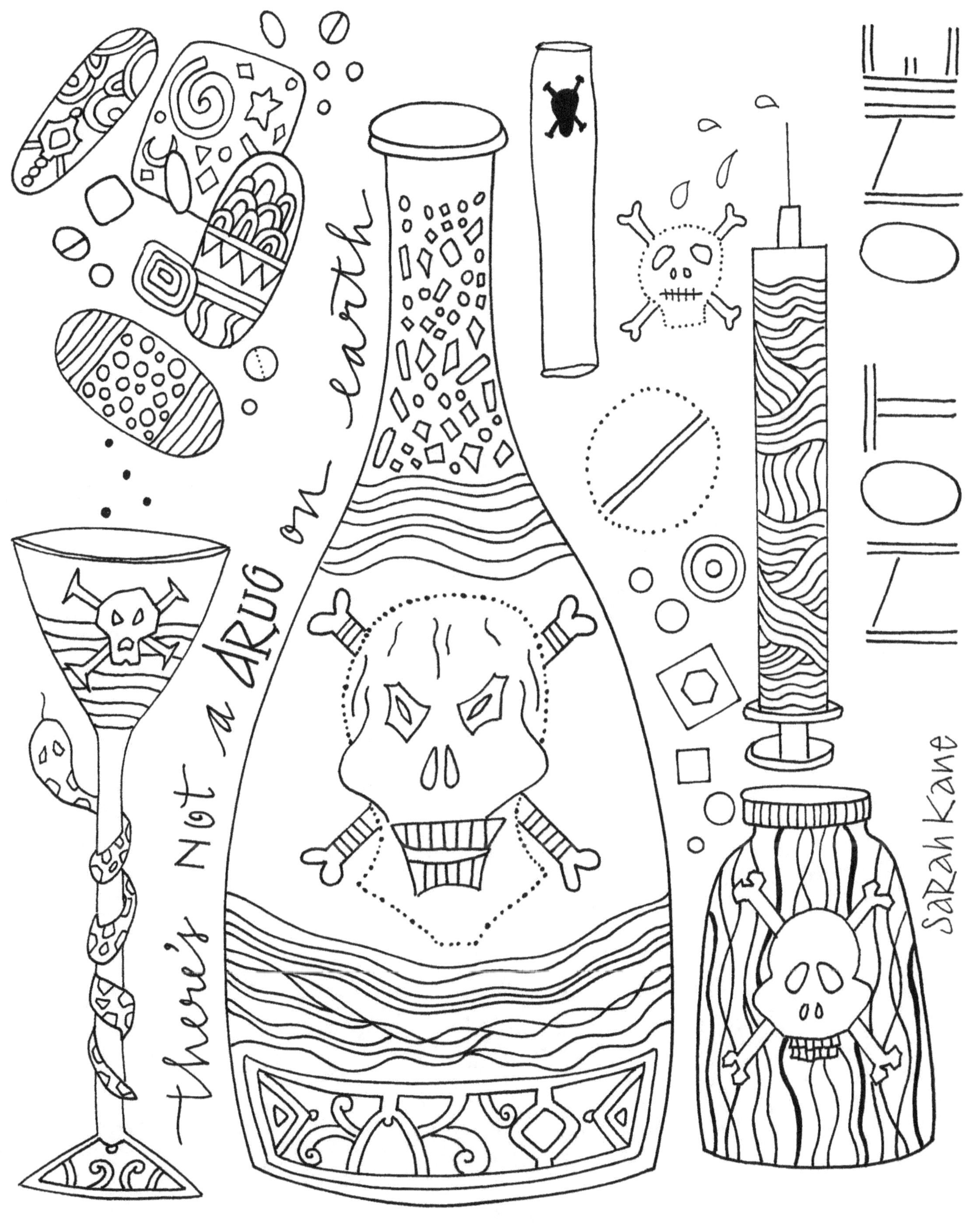
there's Not a dRuG on earth
NOT ONE
Sarah Kane
that can make YOUR LIFE MEANINGFUL

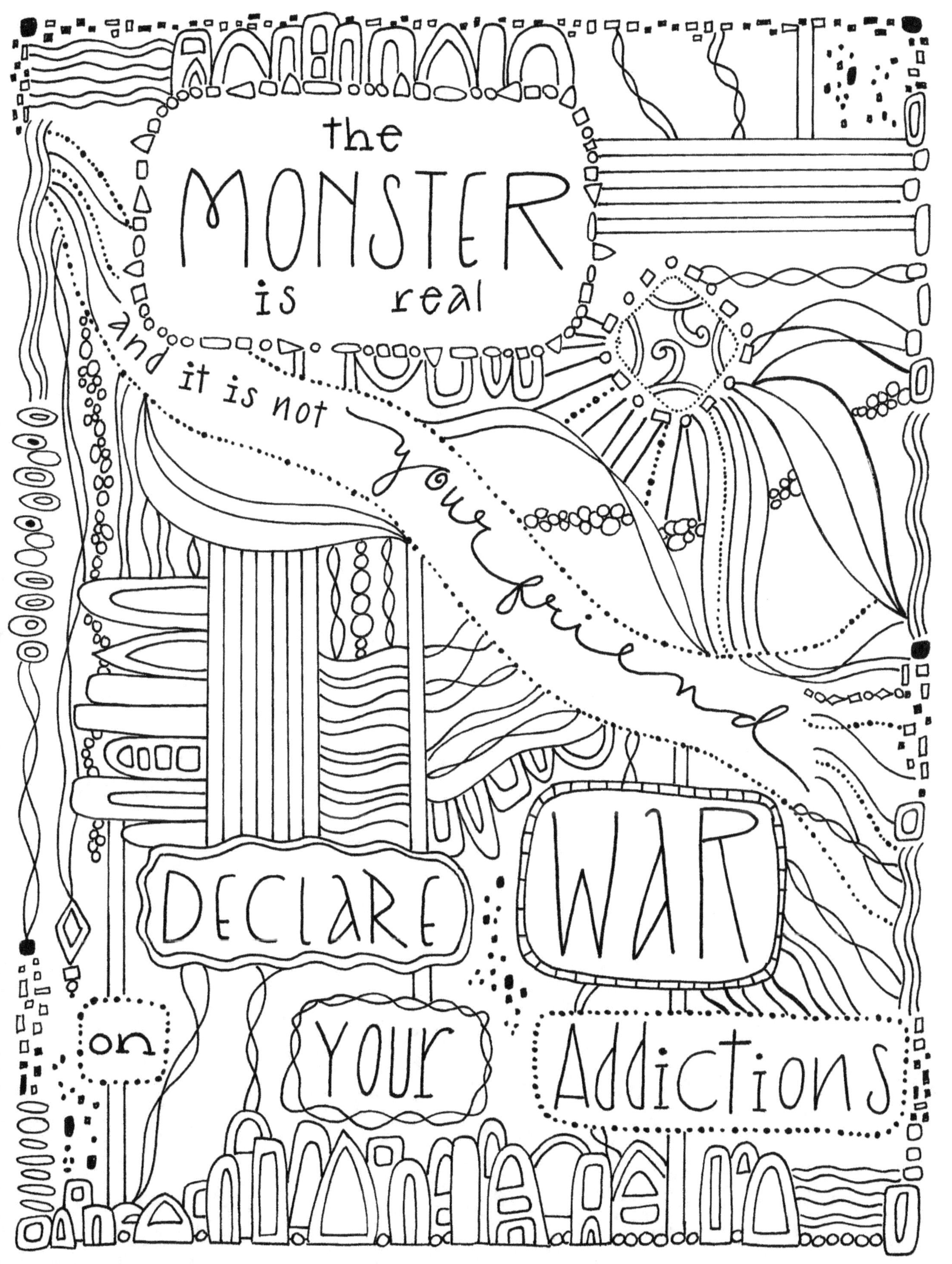

the MONSTER is real
and it is not your friend
DECLARE
on
YOUR
WAR
Addictions

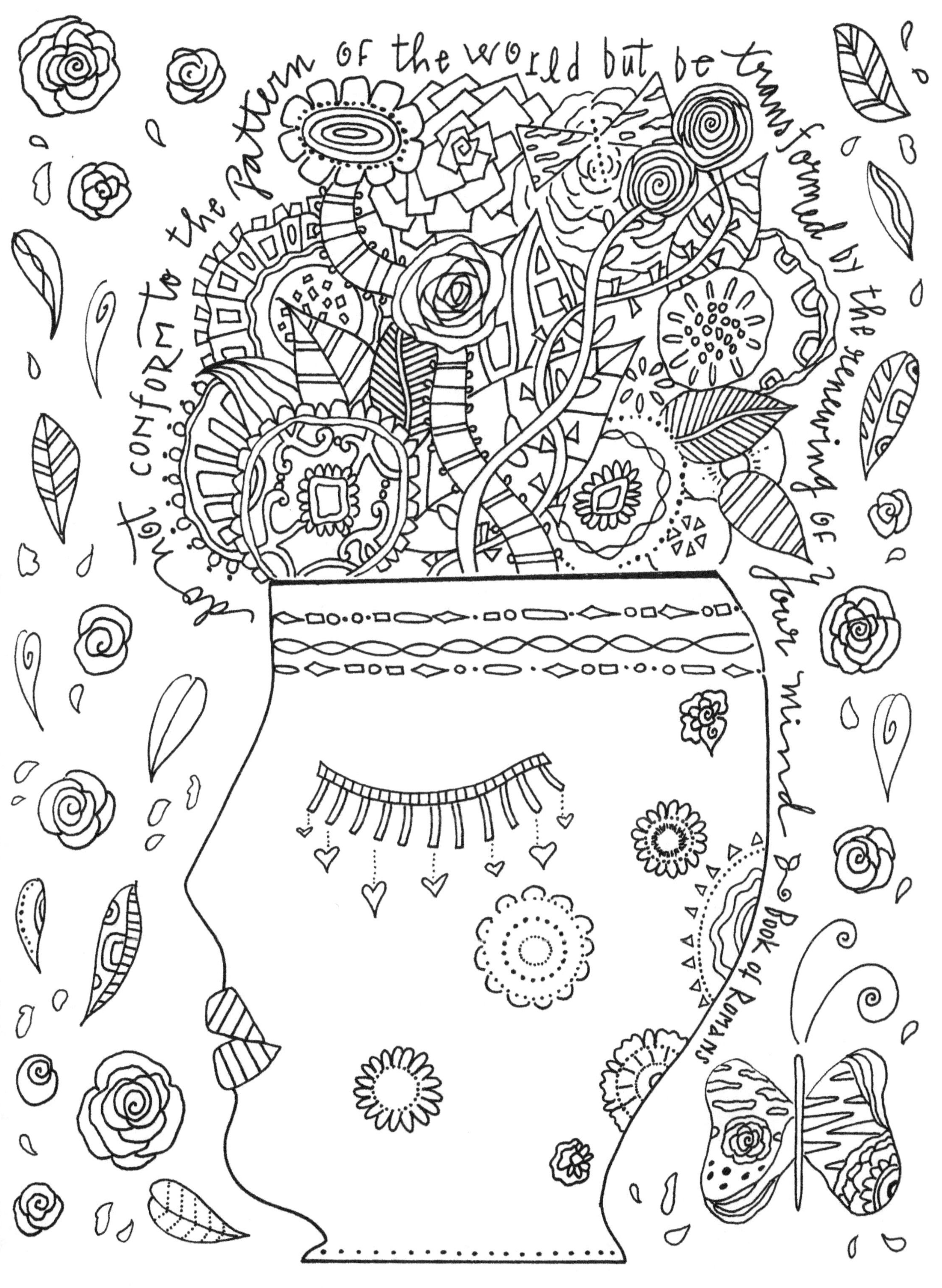

to conform to the pattern of the world but be transformed by the renewing of your mind
Book of Romans

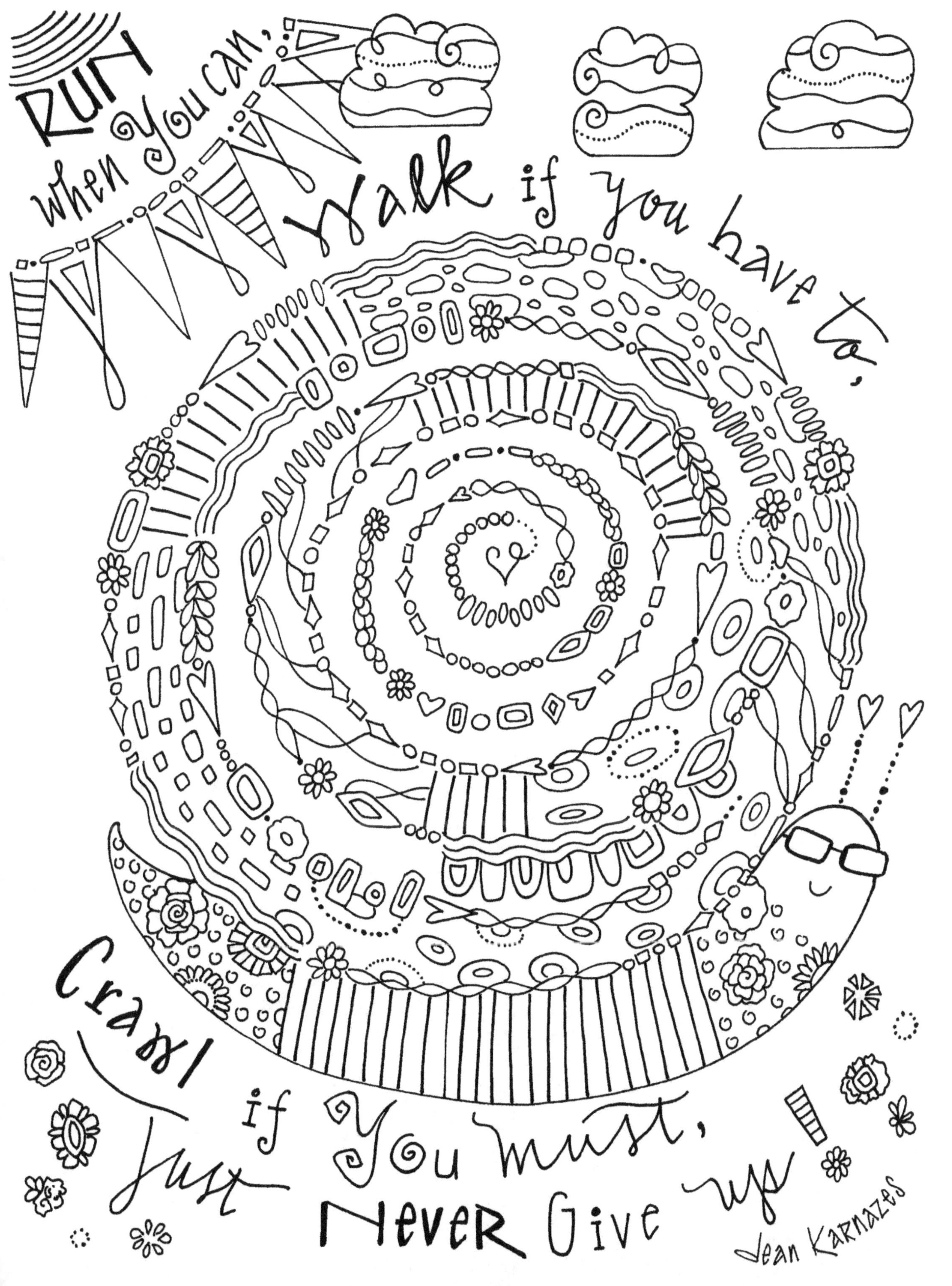

RUN when you can,
Walk if you have to,
Crawl if you must,
Just Never Give up
Dean Karnazes

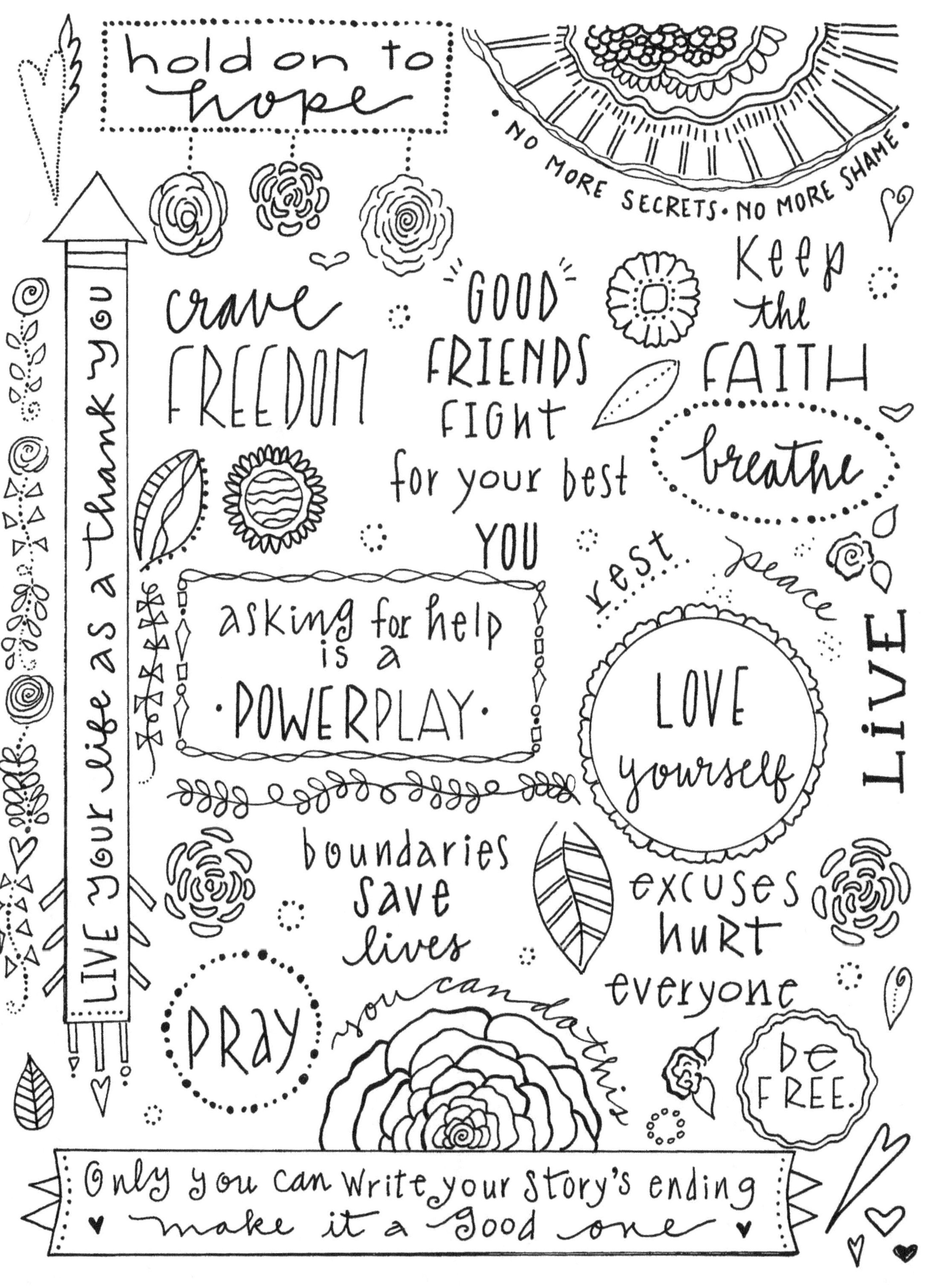

hold on to hope
NO MORE SECRETS · NO MORE SHAME
crave FREEDOM
GOOD FRIENDS FIGHT for your best YOU
KEEP the FAITH
breathe
LIVE your life as a thank you
asking for help is a POWERPLAY·
rest.
peace
LOVE yourself
LIVE
boundaries save lives
excuses huRt everyone
PRAY
you can do this
be FREE.
Only you can write your story's ending
make it a Good one

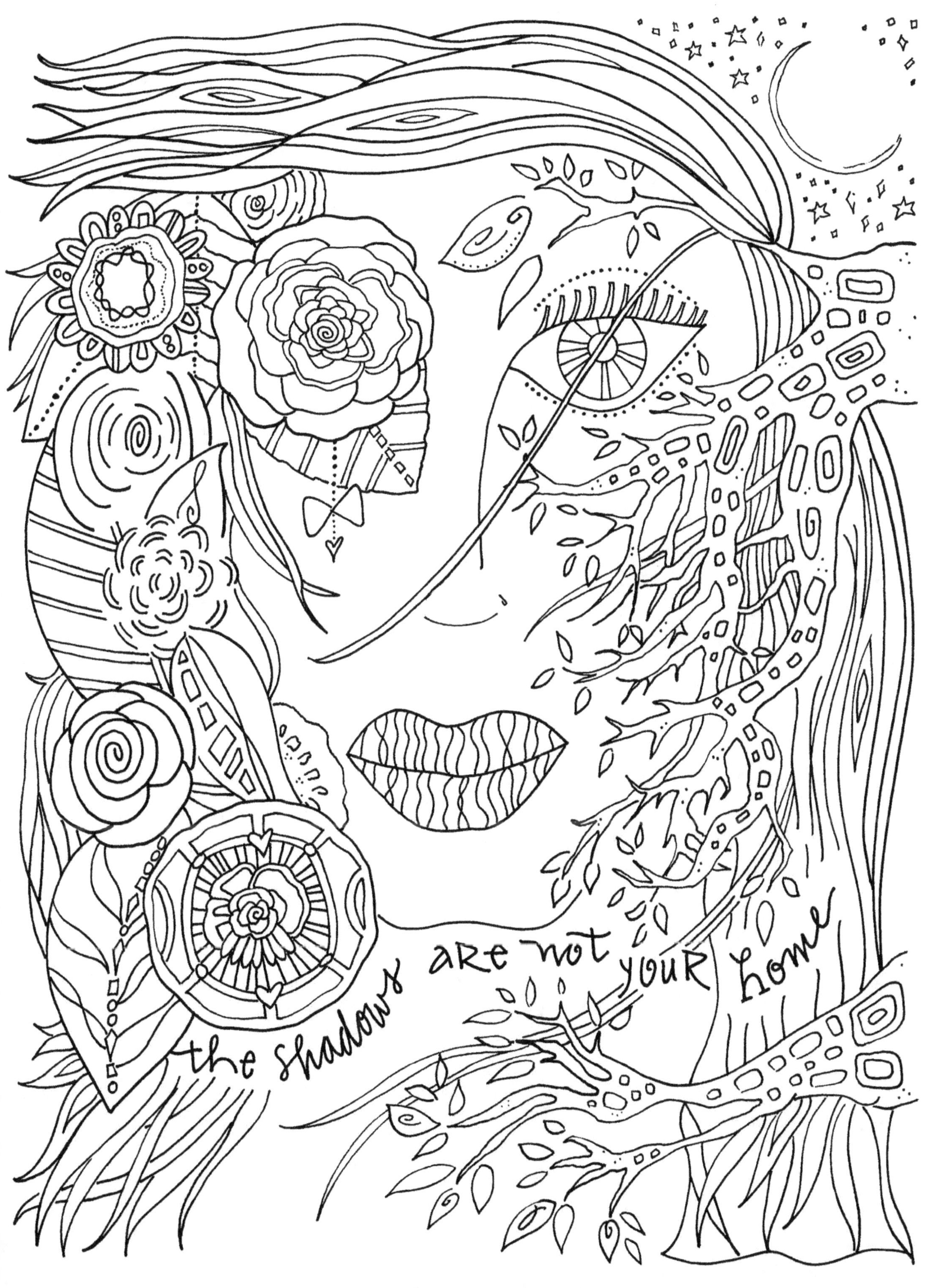

the shadows are not your home

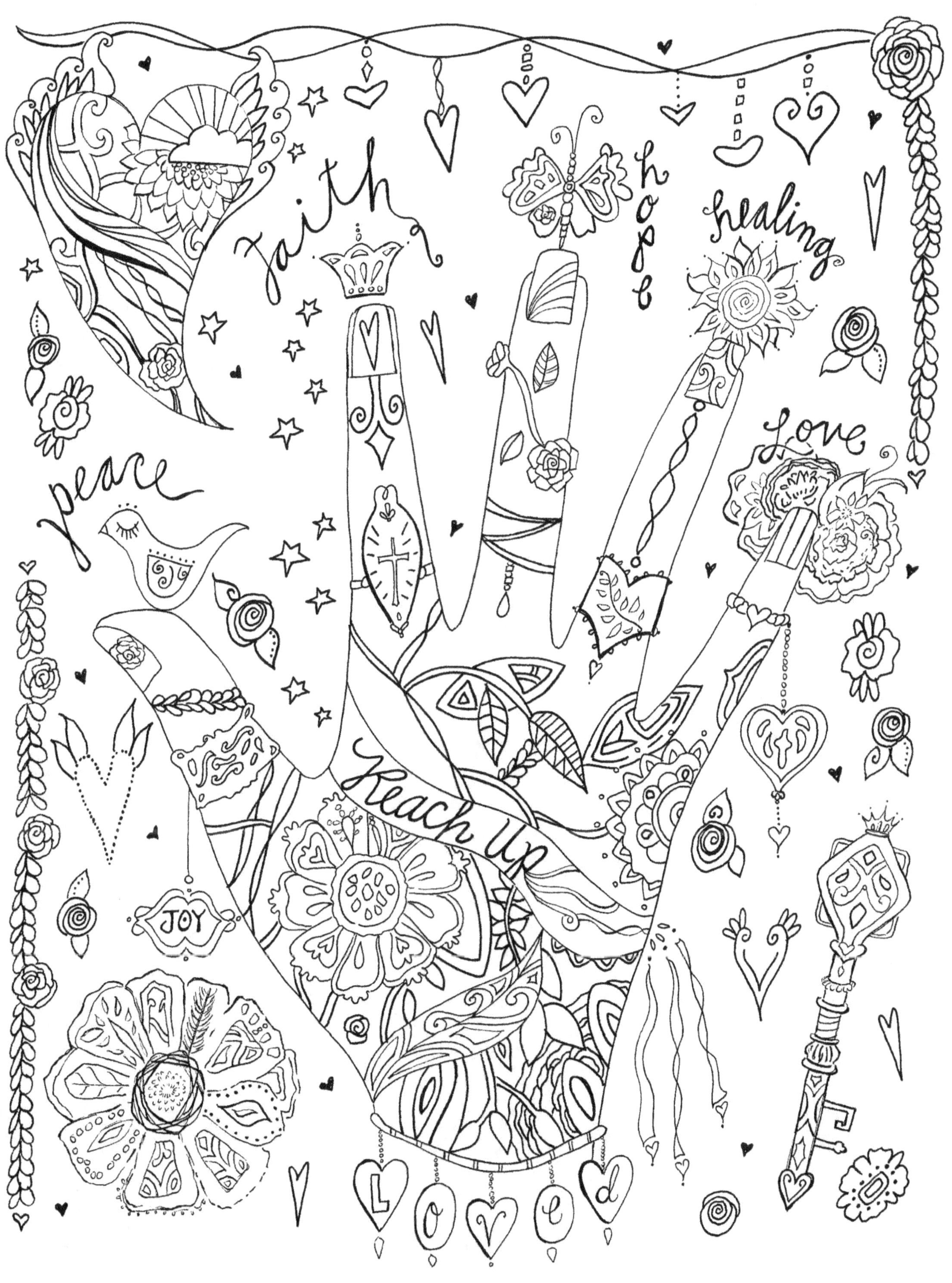

faith
hope
healing
peace
Love
JOY
Reach Up
LOVED

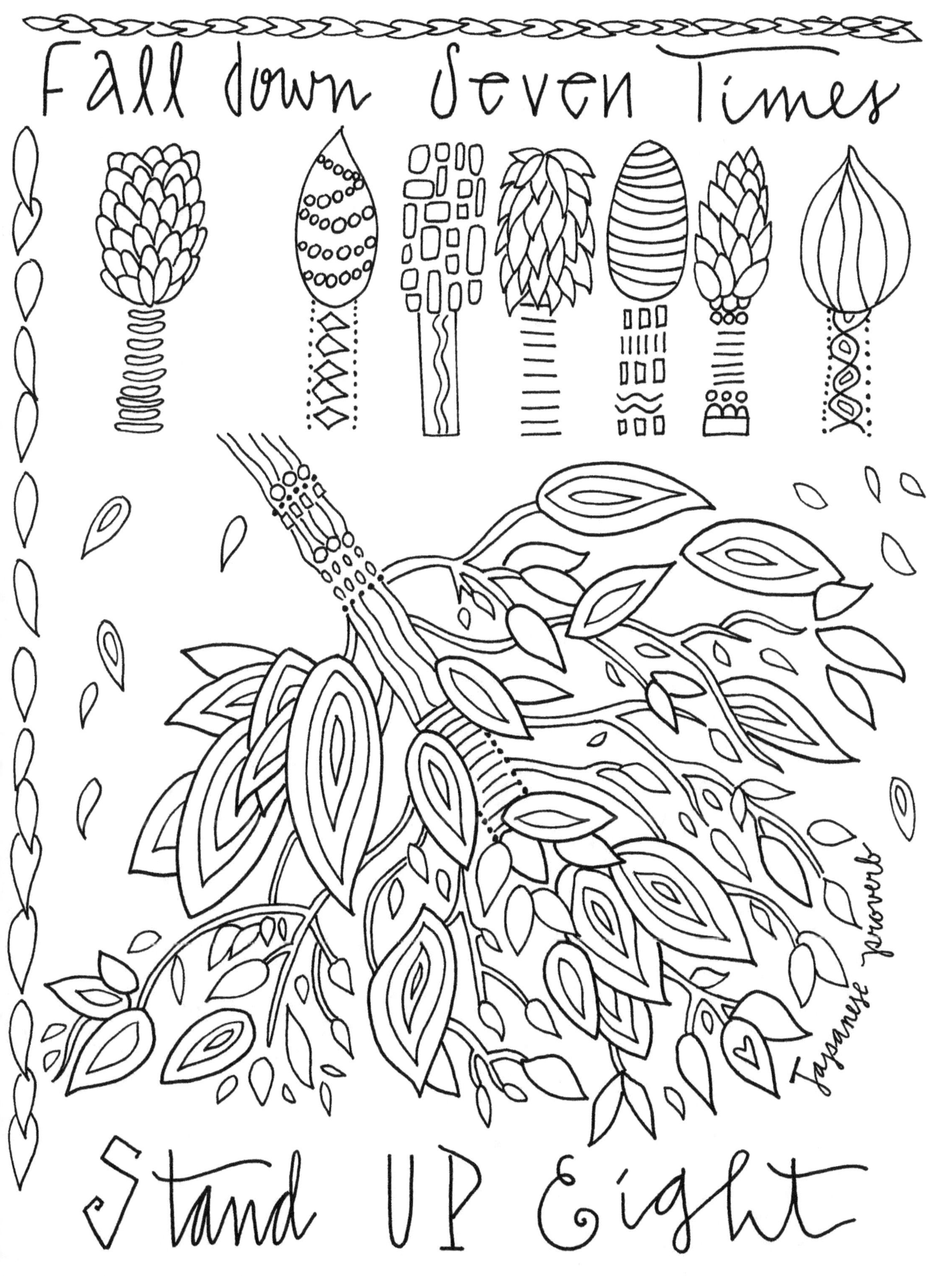

Fall down Seven Times
Stand UP Eight
Japanese proverb

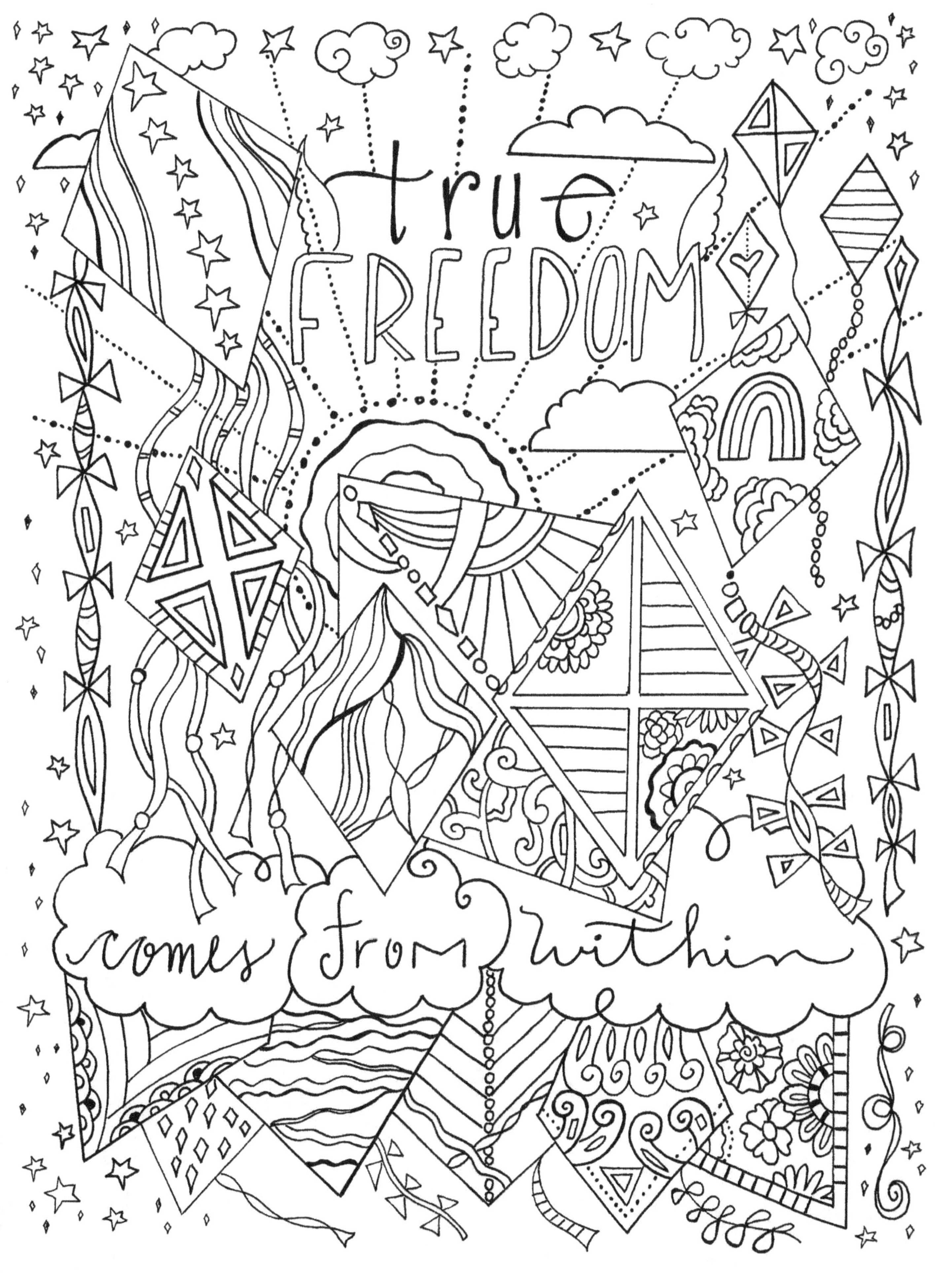

true
FREEDOM
comes from within

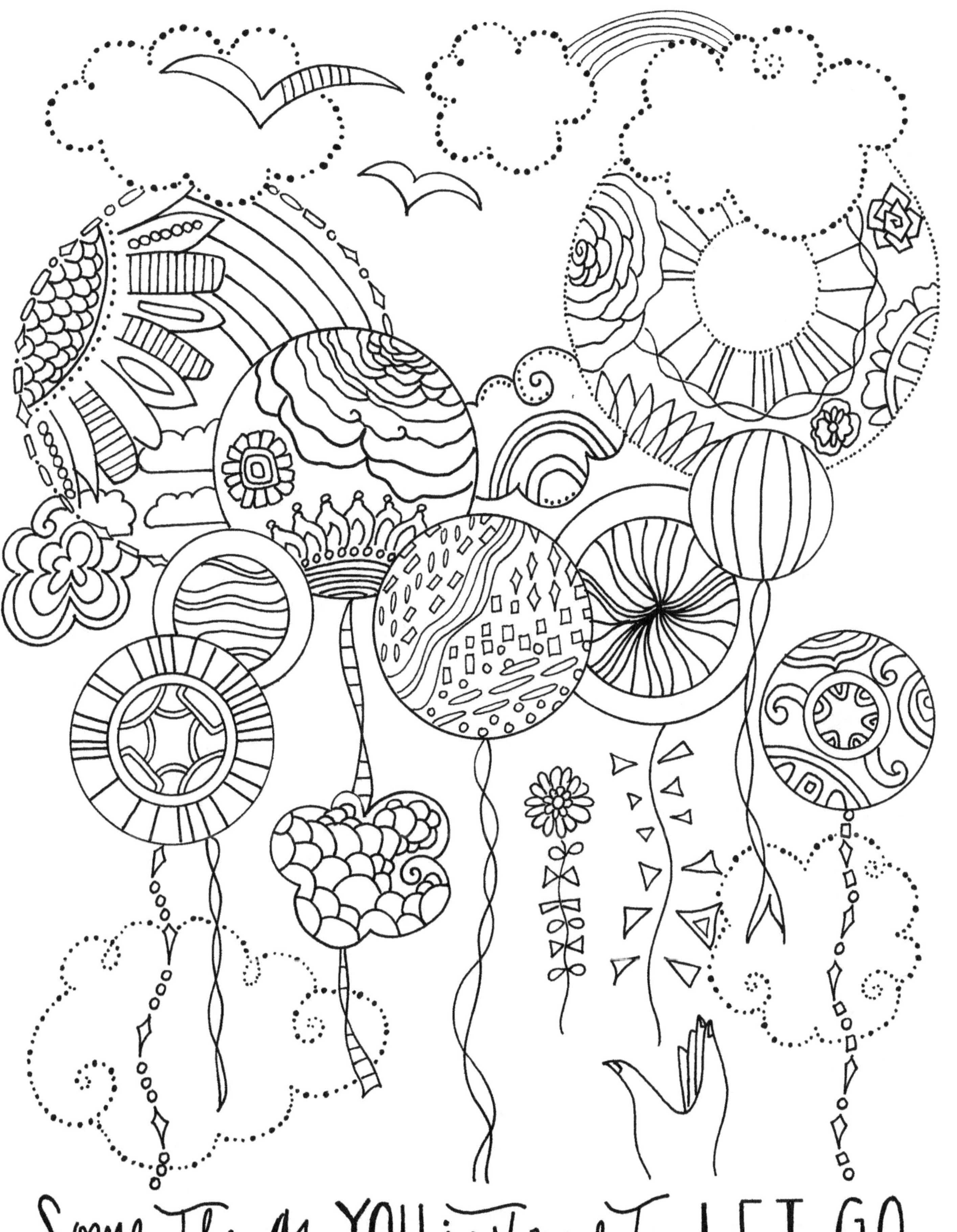

Some things YOU just need to LET GO

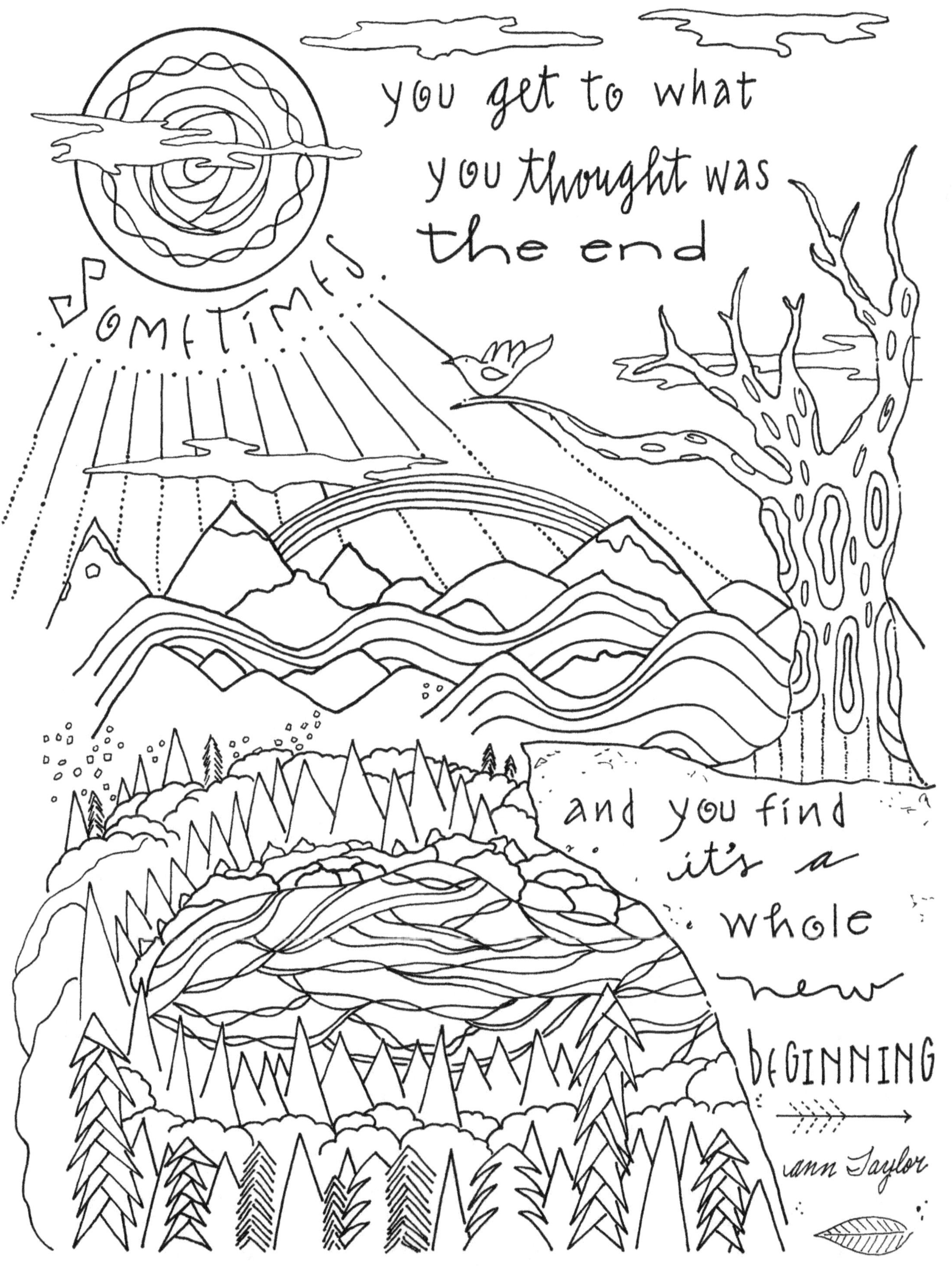

Sometimes...
you get to what you thought was the end
and you find it's a whole new beginning
ann Taylor

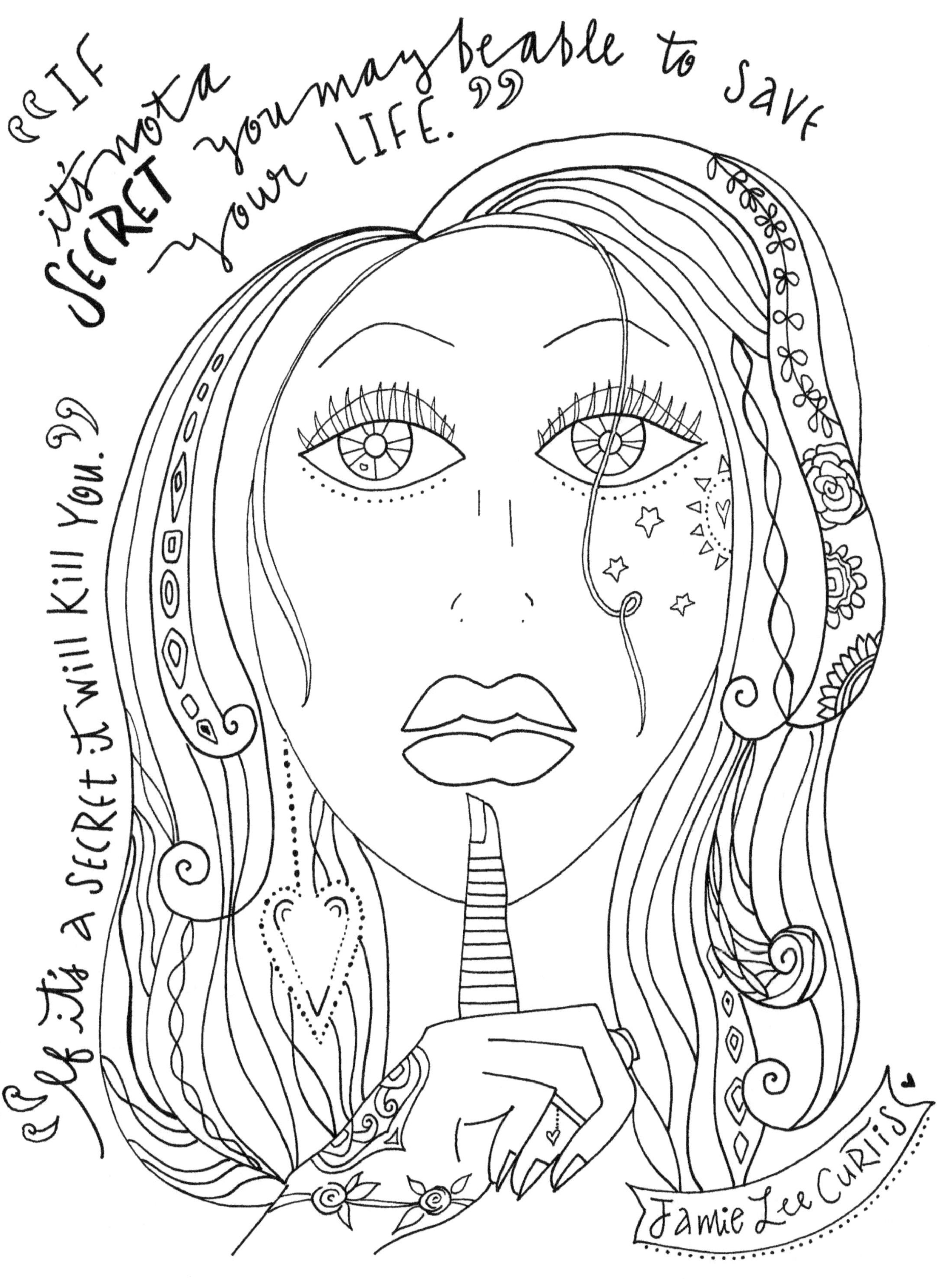

"If it's not a secret you may be able to save your LIFE."
"If it's a secret it will Kill You."
Jamie Lee Curtis

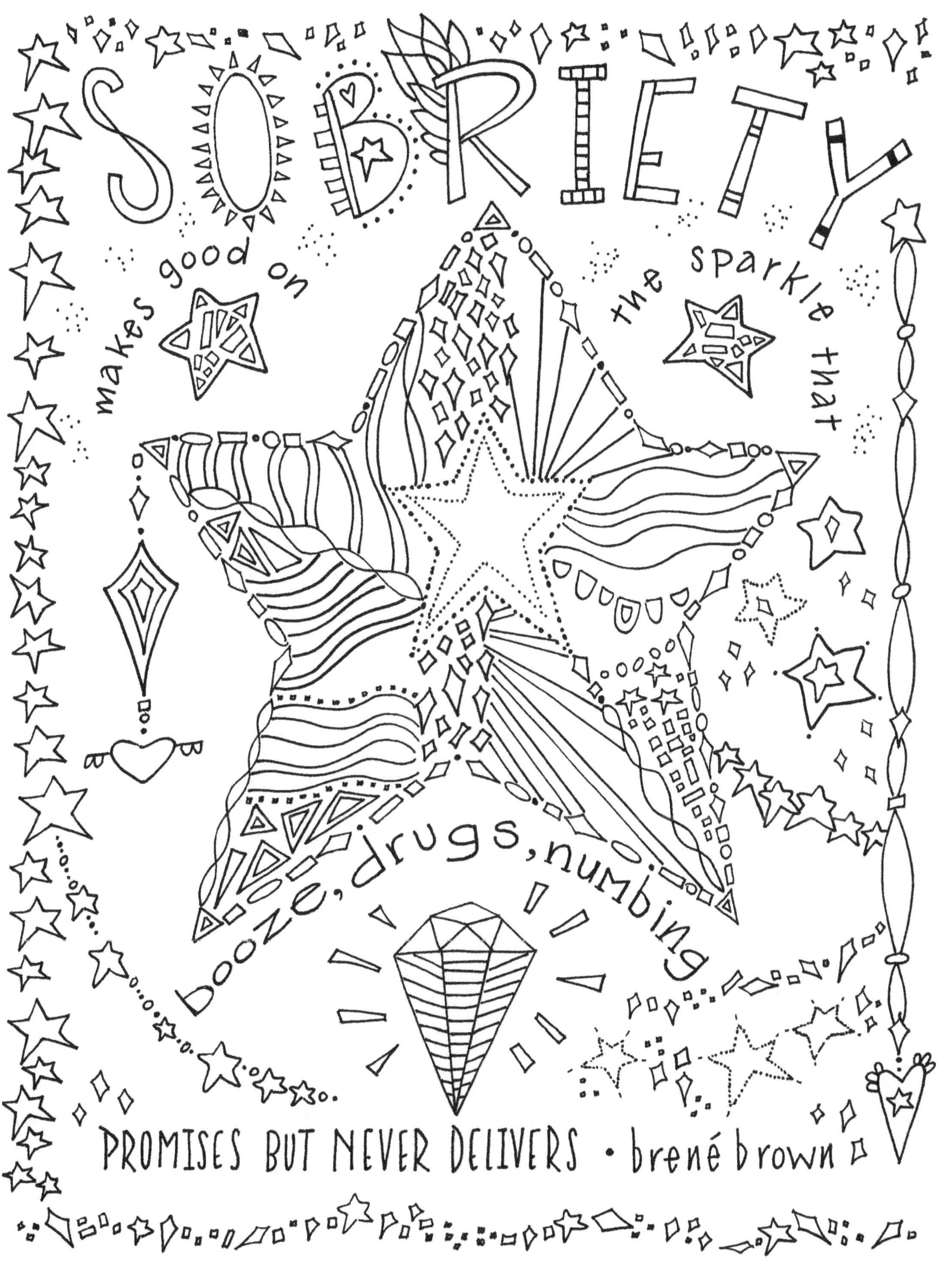

SOBRIETY
makes good on
the sparkle that
booze, drugs, numbing
PROMISES BUT NEVER DELIVERS • brené brown

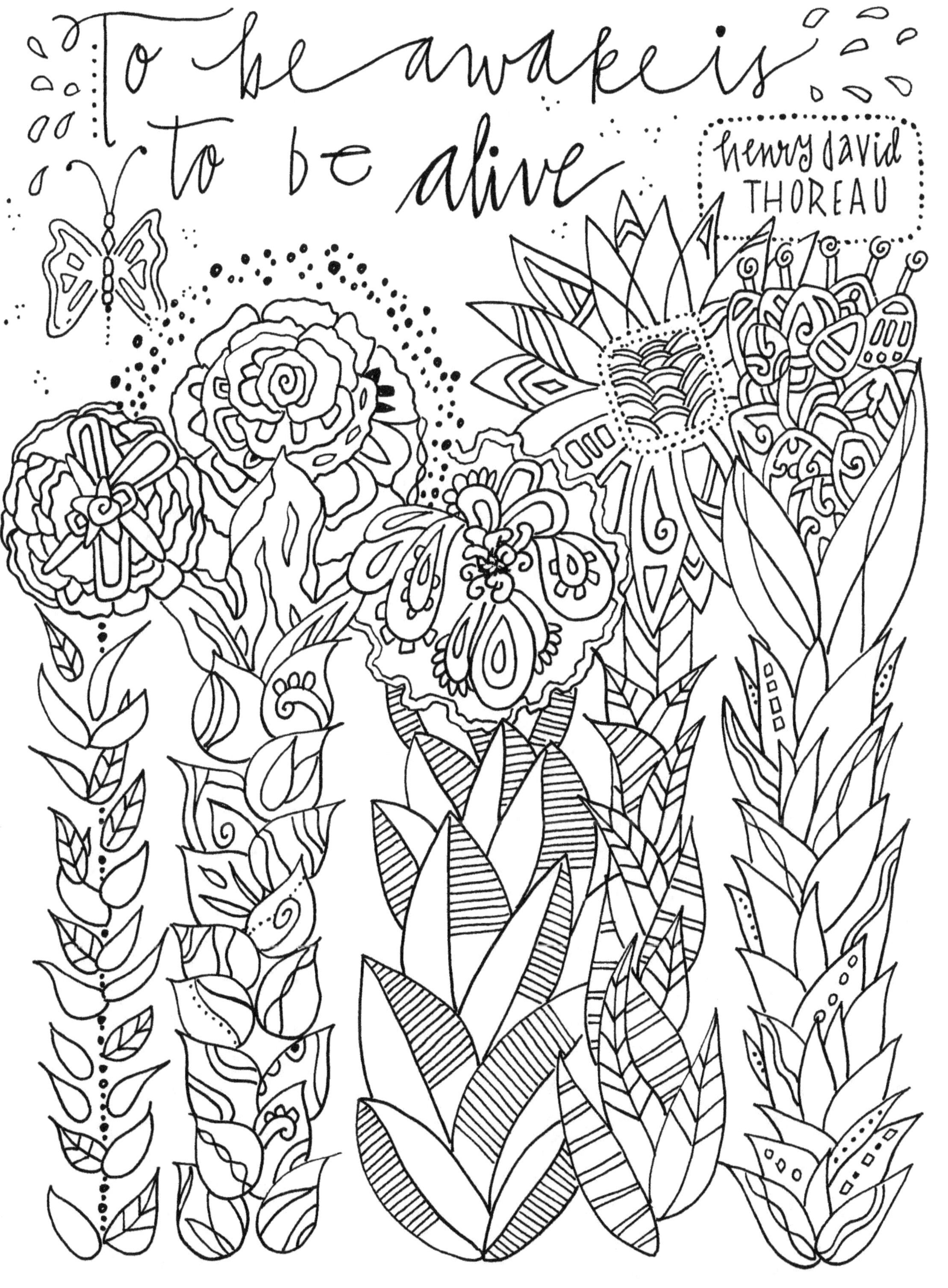

To be awake is to be alive
henry david THOREAU

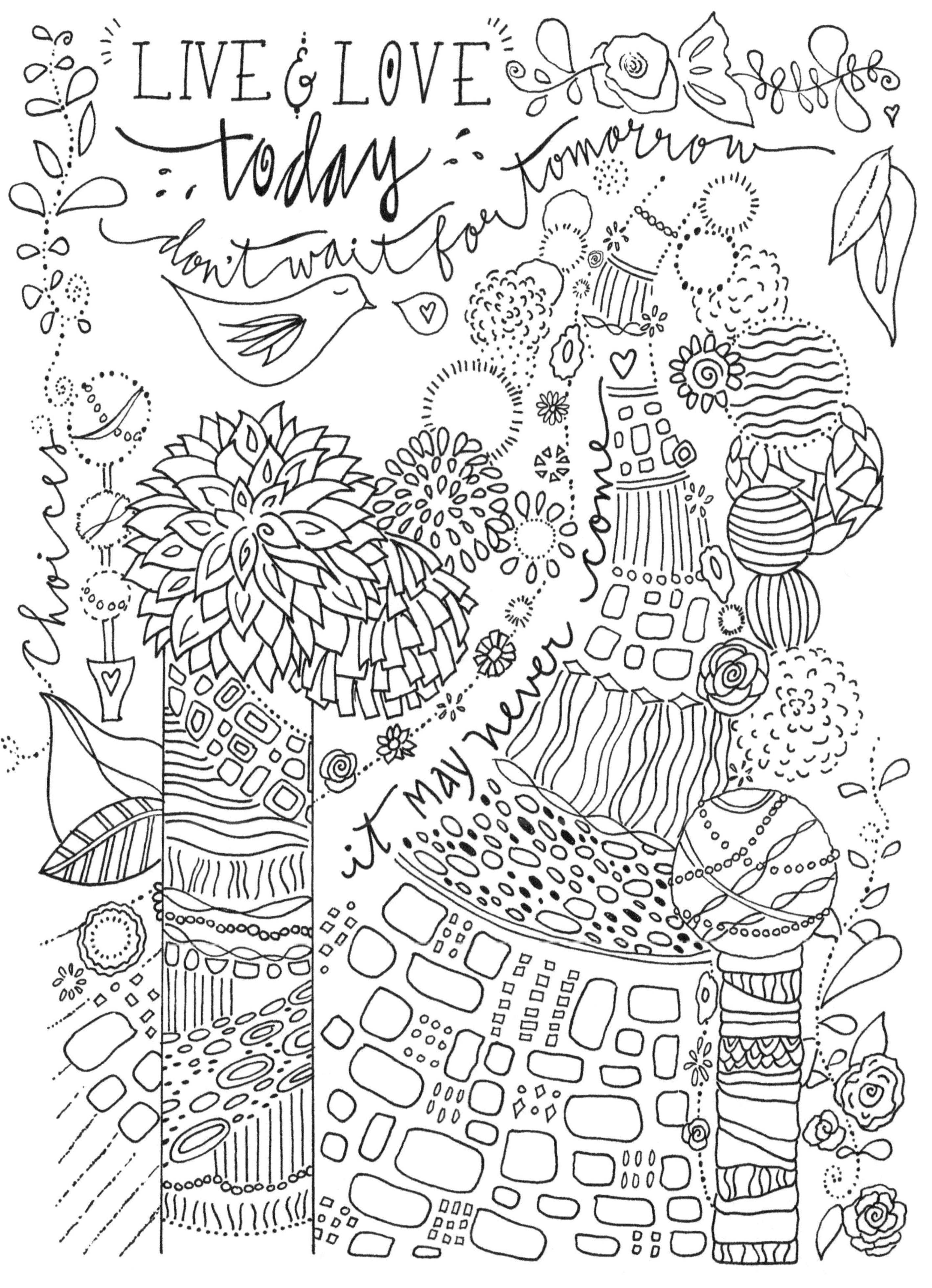

LIVE & LOVE
today
don't wait for tomorrow
it may never come
Choices

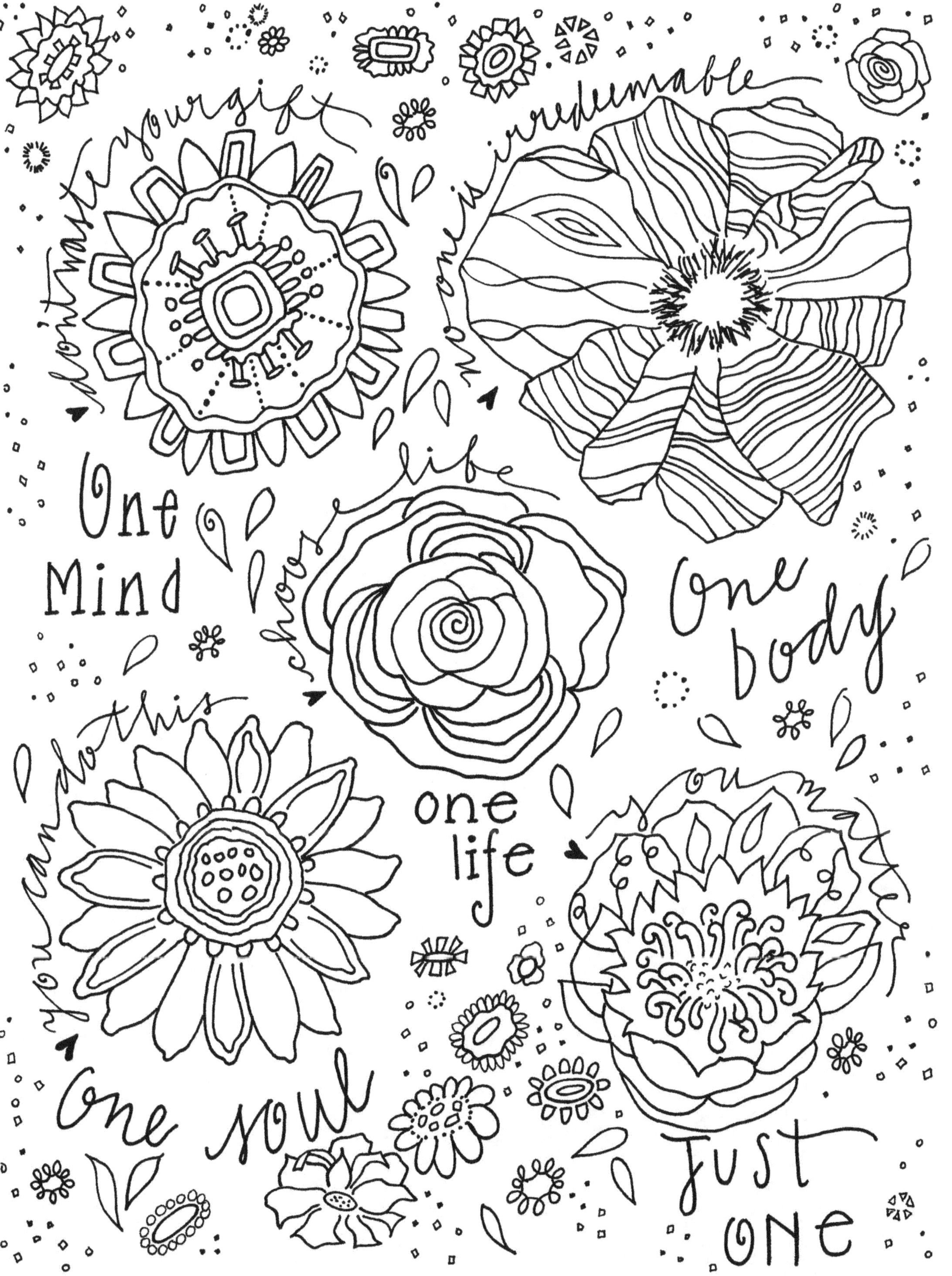
don't waste your gift
no one is irredeemable
One Mind
you can choose life
One body
you can do this
one life
One soul
you
Just one

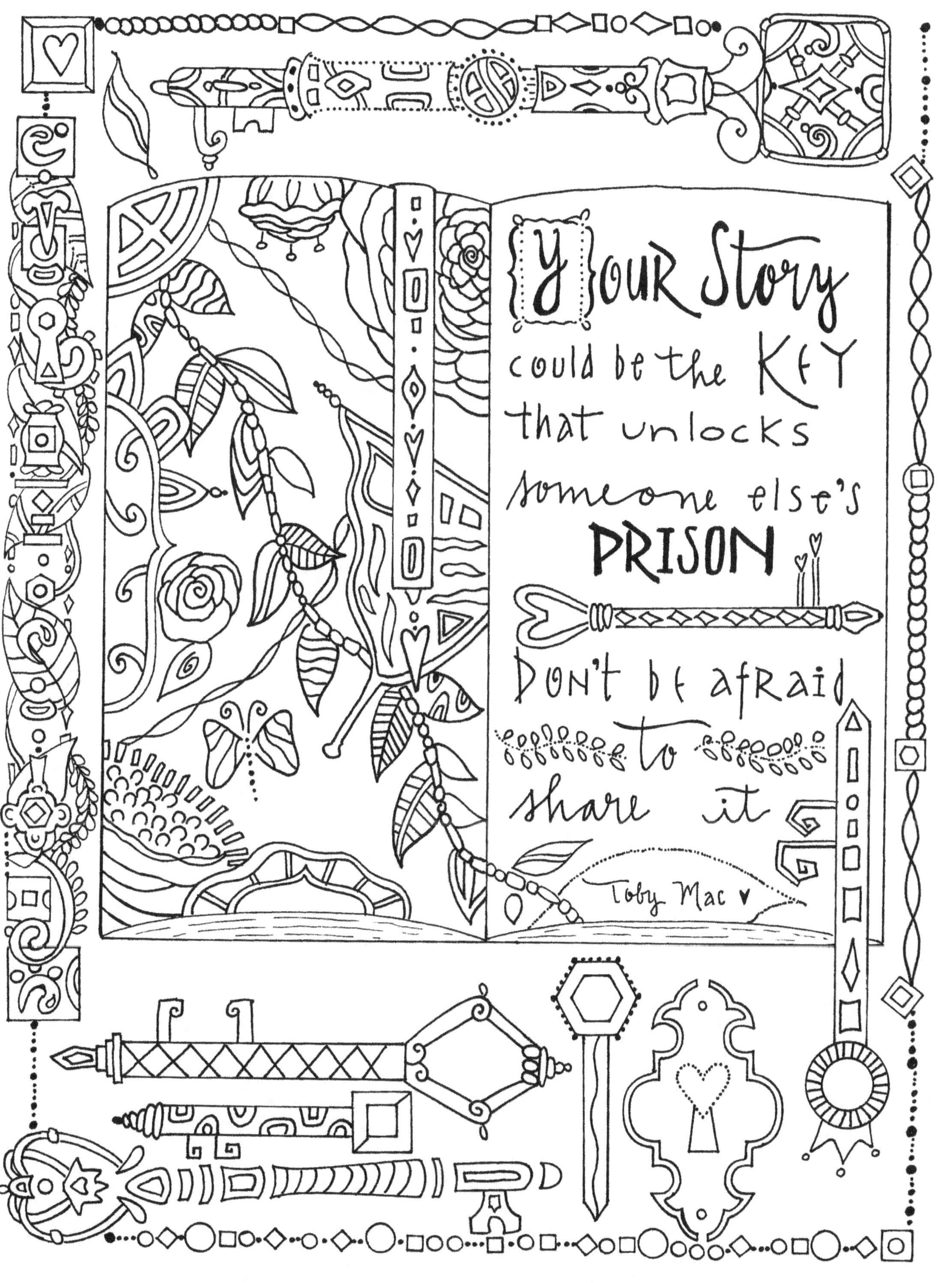

Your Story
could be the KEY
that unlocks
someone else's
PRISON
Don't be afraid
to
share it
Toby Mac

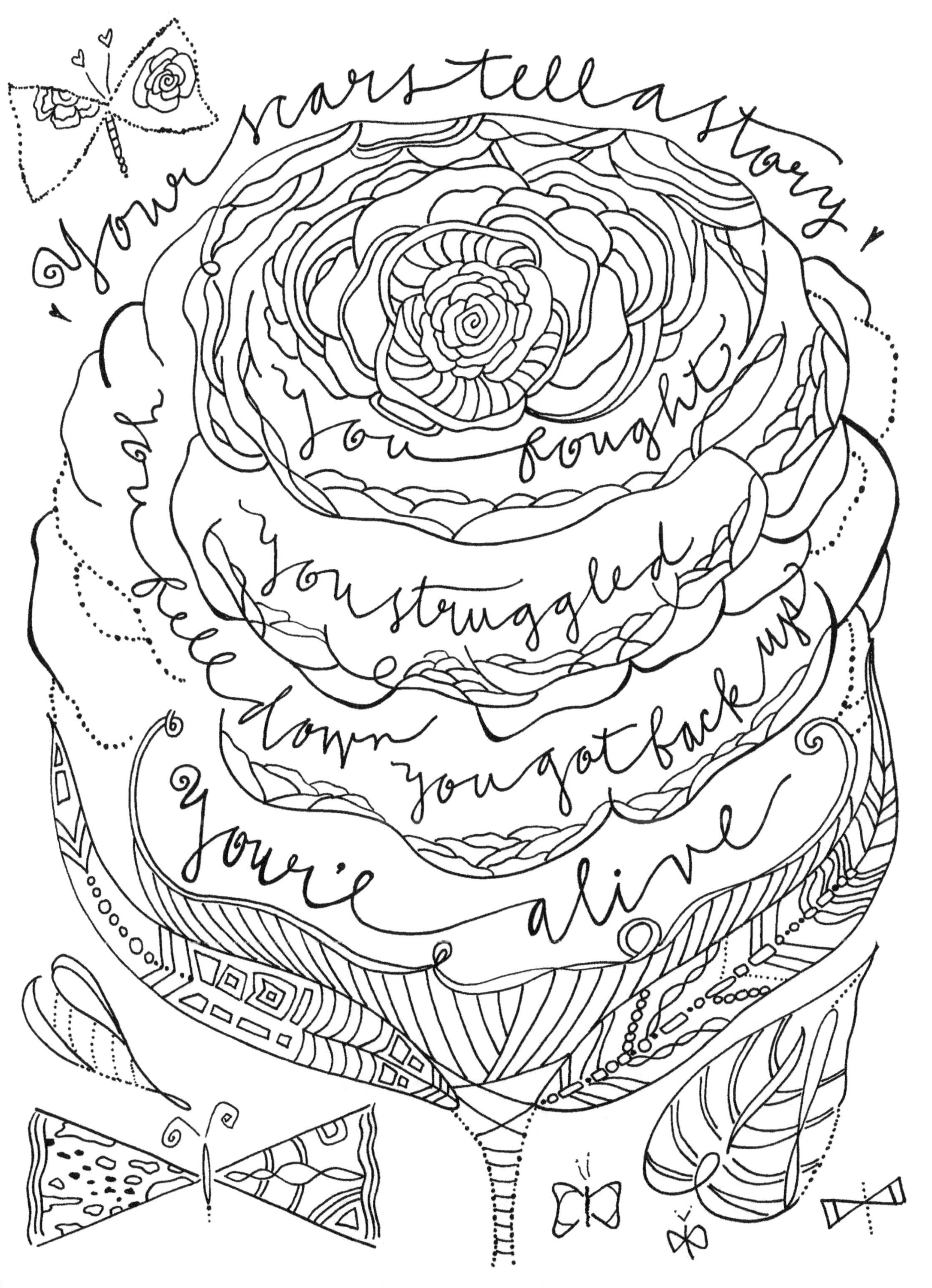
"Your scars tell a story"
You fought
you struggled
fell down you got back up
you're alive

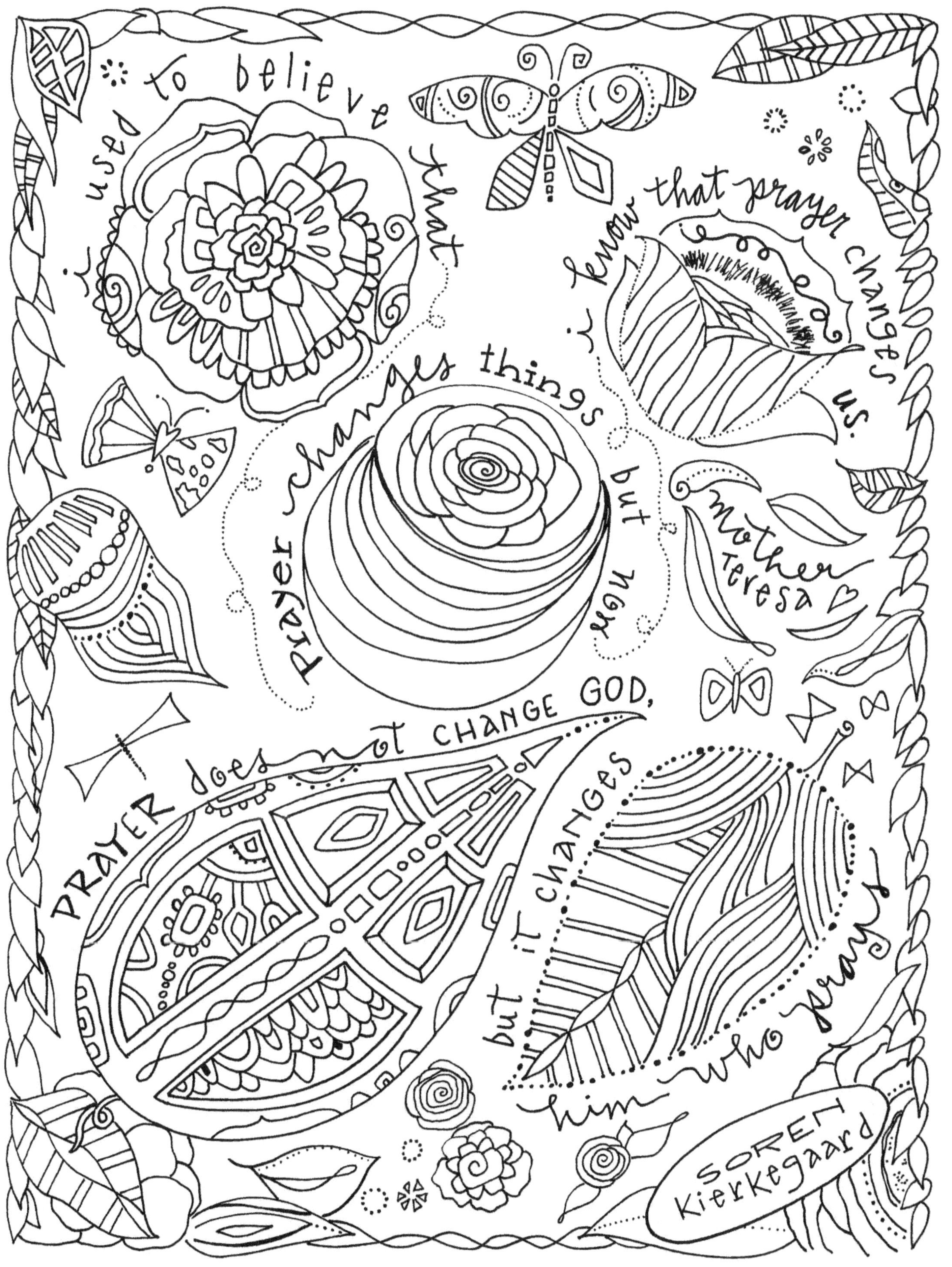
i used to believe that
i know that prayer changes us.
prayer changes things
but now
Prayer changes things
Mother Teresa
Prayer does not change God,
but it changes
him who prays.
Soren Kierkegaard

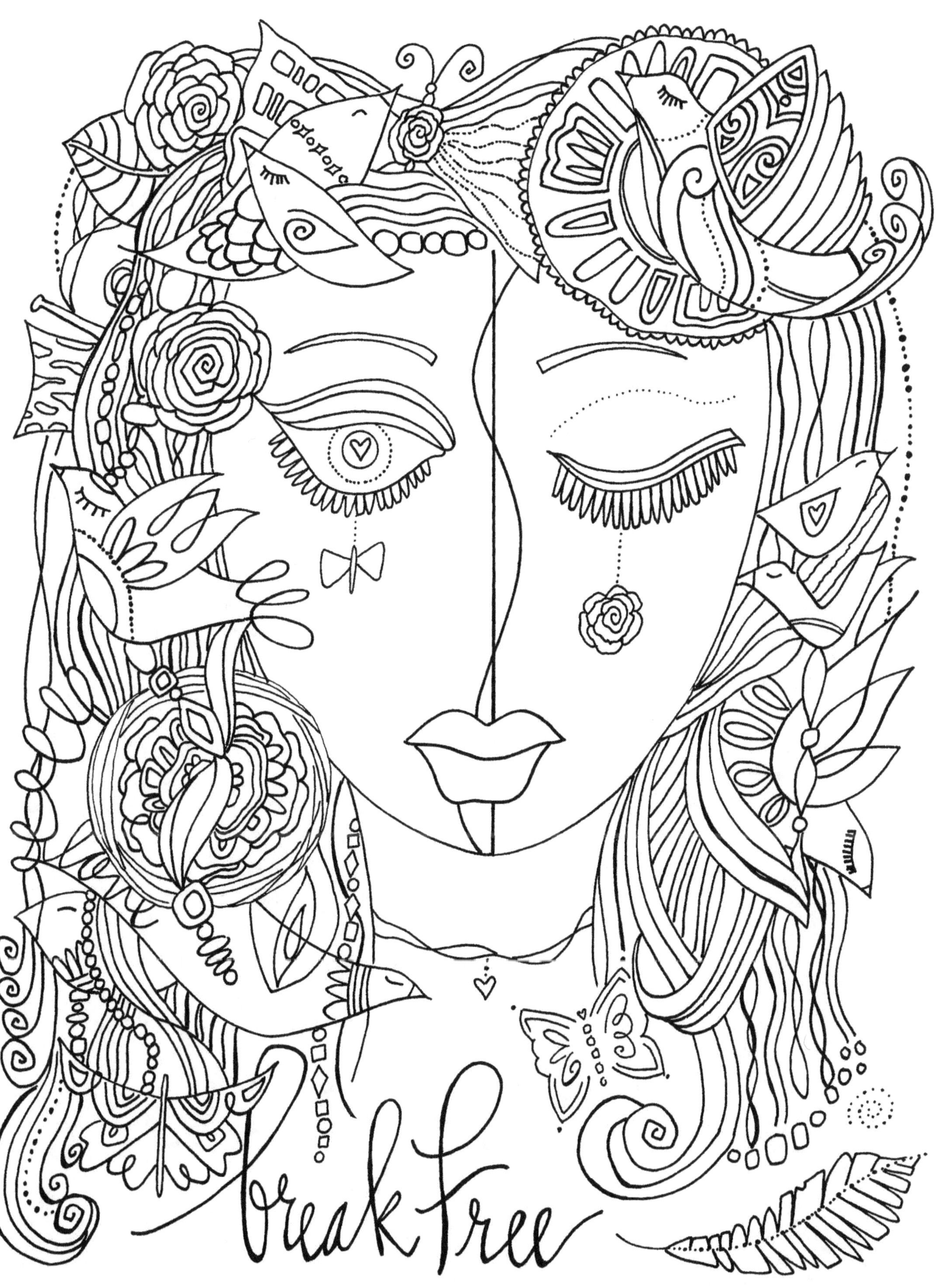
break free

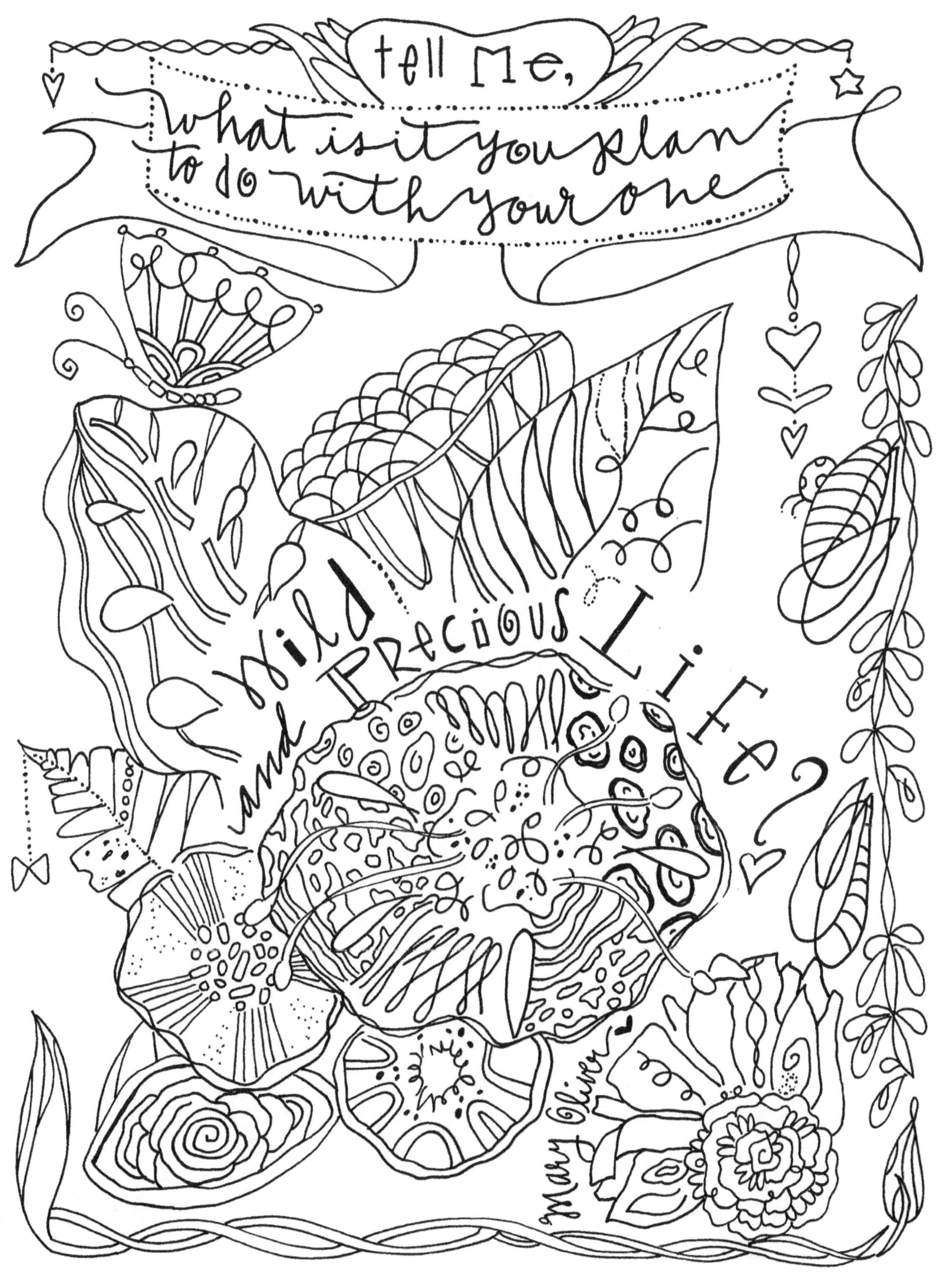

tell me,
what is it you plan
to do with your one
wild and Precious Life?
Mary Oliver

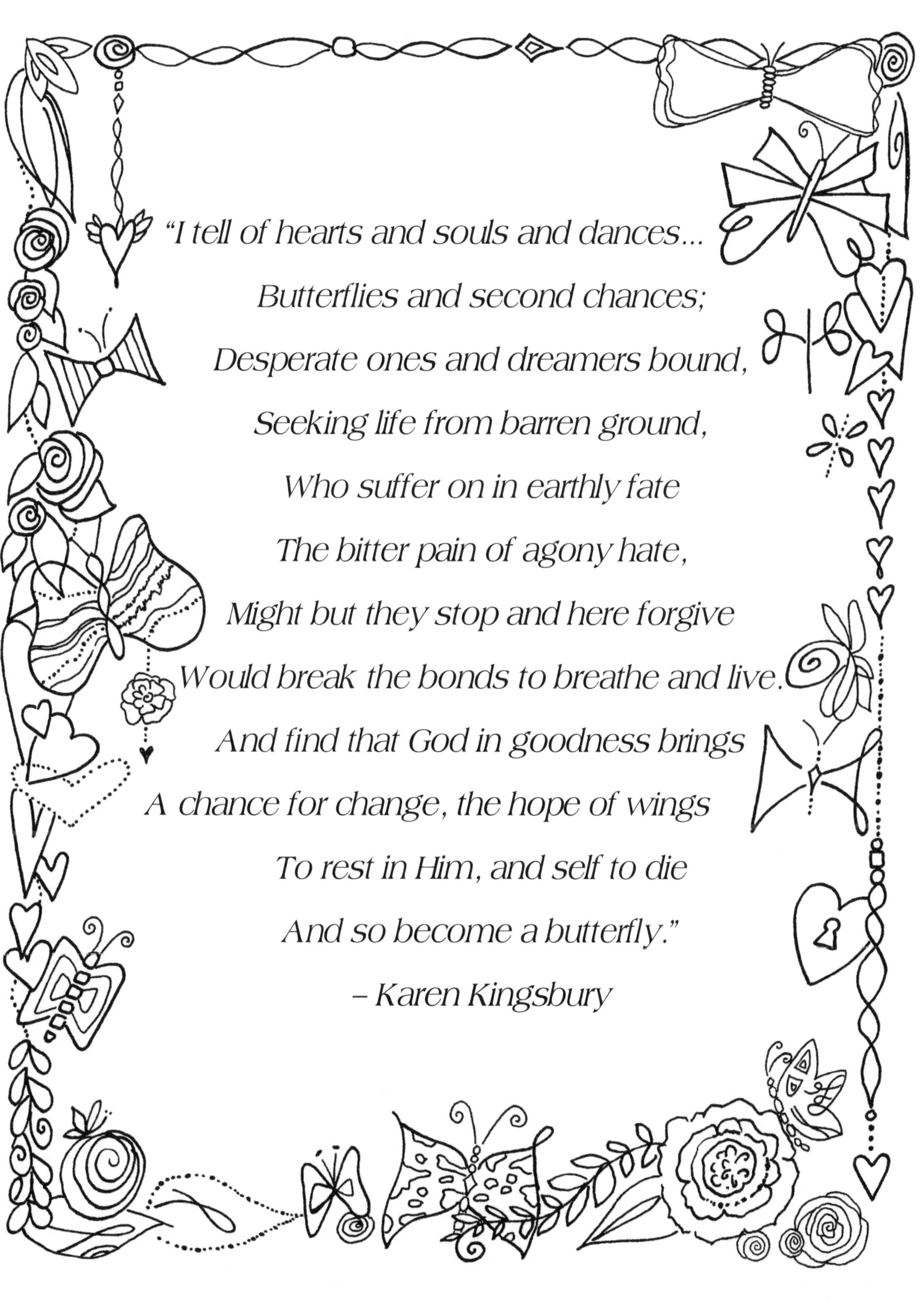

"I tell of hearts and souls and dances...

Butterflies and second chances;

Desperate ones and dreamers bound,

Seeking life from barren ground,

Who suffer on in earthly fate

The bitter pain of agony hate,

Might but they stop and here forgive

Would break the bonds to breathe and live.

And find that God in goodness brings

A chance for change, the hope of wings

To rest in Him, and self to die

And so become a butterfly."

– Karen Kingsbury

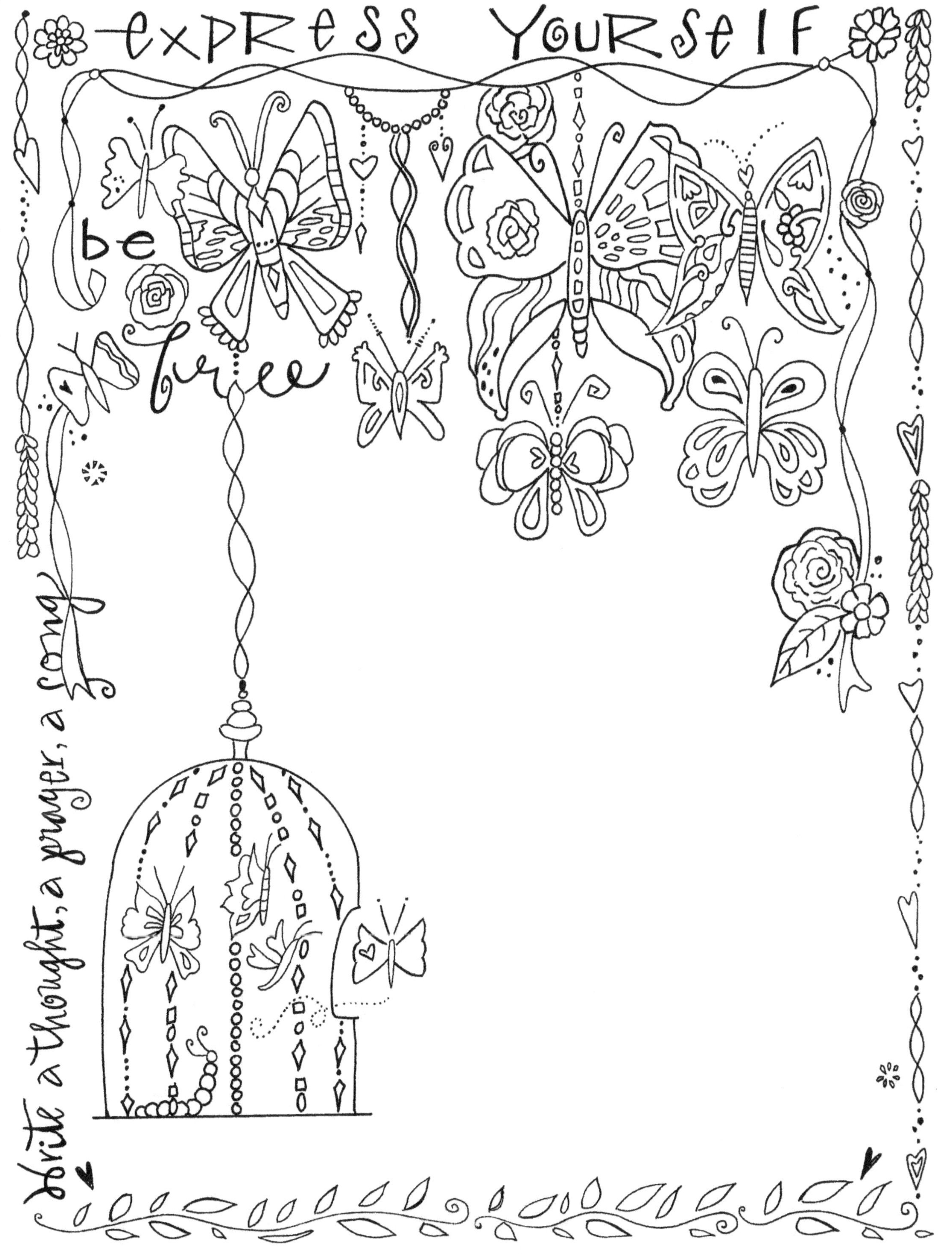

express Yourself
be free
Write a thought, a prayer, a song

# PRACTICE PAGE

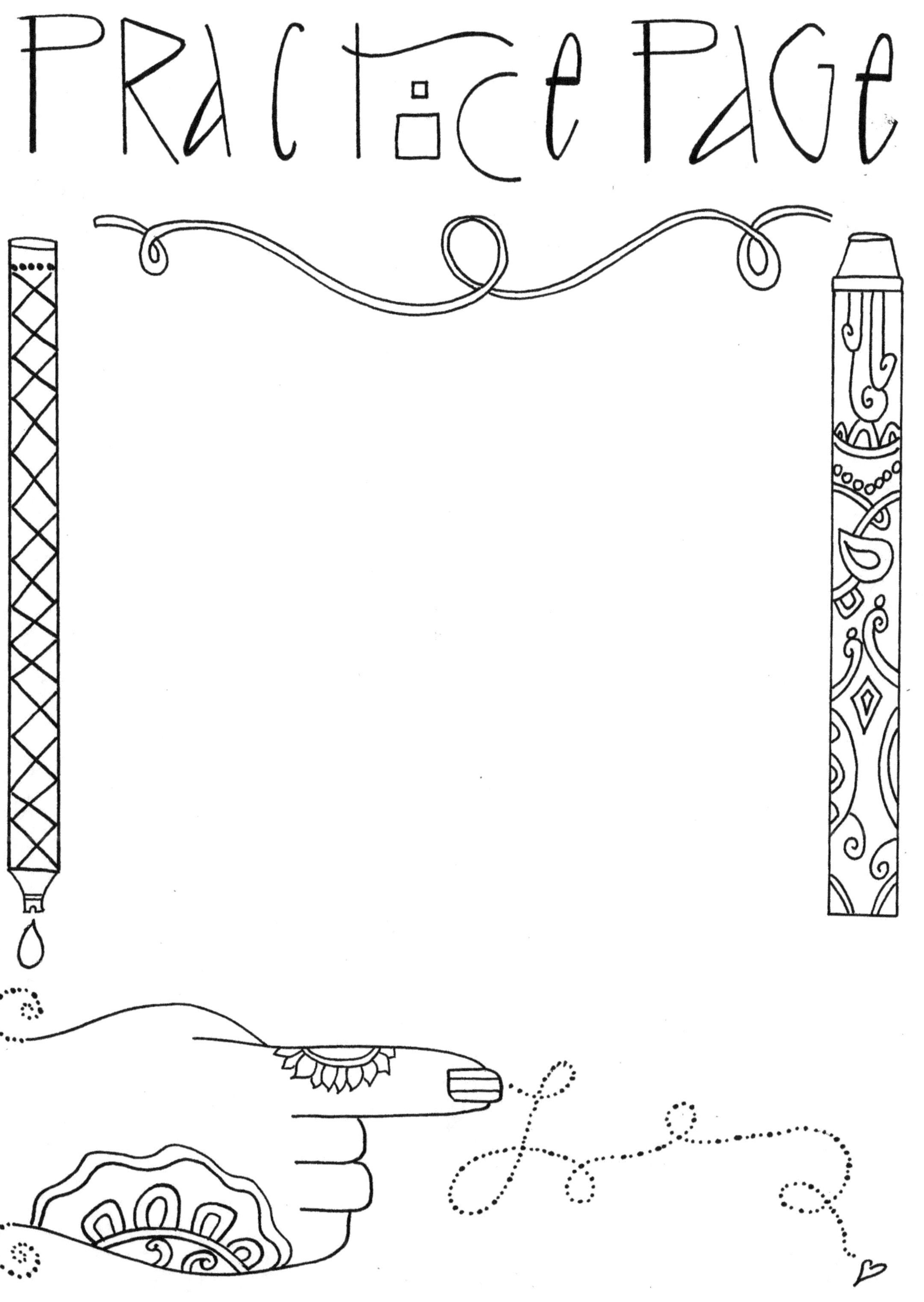

# A Little About April...

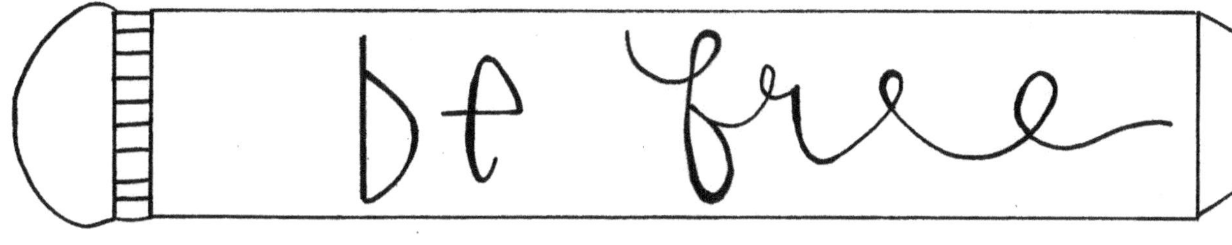


**April McCallum** is an illustrator, cartoonist and writer. Since retiring from a successful career in the high-tech industry, she's focused her creative passions on art, writing and advocacy projects. Her artwork has been licensed and featured on magazine covers, for business and non-profits, and on a variety of gift products. Her writing and artwork has appeared in a variety of magazines and featured on CNBC. Her signature style combines words and visuals, bold color and intricate design. Her writing and illustration work is inspirational, hope-filled and empowering, while her cartoonist side brings a unique twist of humor to the table.

April has long been an advocacy artist designing creative pieces that interweave words and visuals to speak to issues close to her heart. Current topics include empowering women, addiction, grief and loss, adoption, breast cancer awareness and the power of one.

BREAKING FREE: Coloring Book Therapy for Addiction & Recovery
KISS OF LIFE: A Coloring Book to Celebrate Life & Adoption
BRAVE WINGS: A Coloring Book to Celebrate & Empower Women
REFLECTIONS OF LOVE: Coloring Book Therapy for Grief & Loss
COLORS OF HOPE: Breast Cancer Warriors Coloring Book

Pete Berg and April McCallum have been creative collaborators on a variety of colorful and interesting projects over the years. If you would like to connect with Pete Berg regarding a graphic art project, he can be reached at: ohberg3@gmail.com.

Website:    www.aprilmccallumdesigns.com
Email:      april@aprilmccallumdesigns.com
Blog:       DestinysWomen.com
Facebook:   @AprilMcCallumDesigns
Instagram:  @AprilCartoons | @AprilLovesColor | @PinkCartoons
Pinterest:  https://www.pinterest.com/aprilmccallum/

*"Life doesn't get easier or more forgiving, we get stronger and more resilient."*
*— Steve Maraboli*